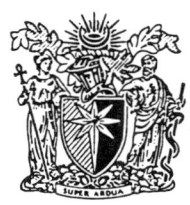

Royal College of Obstetricians and Gynaecologists

LOGIC

SECOND SERIES

Volume 2

Gynaecology

Answer Book

A CME exercise

First published 1995

© Royal College of Obstetricians and Gynaecologists 1995

ISBN 0-902331-72-8 (2-book set)

Published by the **RCOG Press** at the
Royal College of Obstetricians and Gynaecologists
27 Sussex Place
Regent's Park
London NW1 4RG

Registered Charity No: 213280

Cover designed by Geoffrey Wadsley
Printed by the Chameleon Press Limited, London SW18 4SG

PREFACE

With the introduction of Continuing Medical Education it is appropriate for there to be a second series of **LOGIC** (Learning in Obstetrics and Gynaecology for In-service Clinicians). The first volume of the second series was related to obstetrics and this volume is concerned with gynaecology. Instead of forming a Task Force and Editorial Board for this series, the first Chairman of the Education Board, Professor V.R. Tindall, wrote directly to recently appointed consultants and members of certain Committees of the College. The response to this request for MCQ questions in obstetrics and gynaecology was excellent and exceeded expectation. The balance and selection of the 100 questions has therefore been somewhat arbitrary for the first two volumes of this new series and due acknowledgement has been made to those whose contributions are included. While the purpose of **LOGIC** is to educate there is sometimes no absolutely 'correct' or 'incorrect' answer and therefore the explanations given with each question cannot necessarily reflect current College thinking or even the present 'state of the art', but more a consensus view.

Each **LOGIC** topic is produced as a two-book set containing a Question Book and an Answer Book. Fellows and Members wishing to participate in the RCOG CME programme will initially be sent the Question Book and a response sheet. Participants often work through the questions in the comfort of their own home and at their own pace using any reference books they choose.

As CME participants, when we have returned our response sheets, we will receive the second package containing the Answer Book with the 'correct' answers and an explanation as to why it was felt to be so and why the alternatives were considered inappropriate. A small number of recent references or appropriate suggestions for further reading will be given with each answer.

Fellows and Members seeking CME credits for work at home may elect to subscribe to any or all of the parts of **LOGIC** but it is hoped that most will feel it worth while to subscribe to each successive part in order to help us keep our postgraduate educational standards up to a high level. The rapid pace of advance over the whole field of obstetrics and gynaecology makes it difficult for busy practising clinicians to keep up to date and the need to be so is emphasised by the growing awareness of the public we serve of what is and what is not modern practice.

Sadly too, this is also reflected in the small, but increasing, number of dissatisfied patients who embark on litigation. As clinicians we all need to give our patients a first-class service based on up-to-date knowledge of the specialty and our own clinical experience. Participants in the CME **LOGIC** series (produced by our own Fellows and Members), with its practical and clinical options, will help us to give as good a service as the constraints of our working conditions allow.

R.D. Atlay
Chairman, CME Committee

CONTRIBUTORS TO LOGIC SECOND SERIES
VOLUME 2: GYNAECOLOGY

The Royal College of Obstetricians and Gynaecologists wishes to thank all those who sent in questions. There was not sufficient space to include every question in this volume but the willing help of all the contributors is gratefully acknowledged.

Mr Peter Bowen-Simpkins
Professor Linda D. Cardozo
Dr Matthew J. Carty
Miss Barbara D. Case
Mr Glyn Constantine
Dr Paul Donnai
Mr Effi Eyong
Mr Graham Foat
Mr Pharic N. Gillibrand
Dr Anna F. Glasier
Professor John Guillebaud
Mr Robert H. Hammond

Miss Leila S.F. Hanna
Mr M. John Hare
Miss Margaret R. Howells
Professor David M. Jenkins
Professor Ian R. Johnson
Mr Geoffrey Lane
Mr Frank G. Lawton
Dr Mary Ann Lumsden
Mr John H. Macdonald
Dr Eamon P.J. McGuinness
Dr Tahir A. Mahmood
Dr Alistair W.F. Miller

Mr John M. Monaghan
Dr Alison P. Murdoch
Professor P.M. Shaughn O'Brien
Mrs Angela Railton
Mr David H. Richmond
Mr Peter G. Saunders
Mr John H. Shepherd
Miss Jane E. Spring
Mr Charles R. Stewart
Mrs Sheila M. Walker
Mr John Webster
Mr Malcolm I. Whitehead

GLOSSARY

AFP	alphafetoprotein		IUD	intrauterine device
ALO	Actinomyces-like organism		IUI	intrauterine insemination
AMF	anti-Müllerian factor		IVF	*in-vitro* fertilisation
APAS	antiphospholid antibody syndrome		KCT	kaolin clotting time
APTT	activated partial thromboplastin time		kHz	kilohertz
b.d.	*bis die* – twice a day		LDL	low density lipoproteins
BMI	body mass index		LH	luteinising hormone
BSO	bilateral salpingo-oophorectomy		LHRH	luteinising hormone releasing hormone
CAH	congenital adrenal hyperplasia		LMP	last monthly period
CI	confidence interval		LNG	levonorgestrel
CIN	cervical intraepithelial neoplasia		LUF	luteinised unruptured follicle
CL	corpus luteum		MESA	microepididymal sperm aspiration
COC	combined oral contraception		mg	milligram
COH	controlled ovarian hyperstimulation		mHz	megahertz
CVD	cardiovascular disease		MRC	Medical Research Council
D&C	dilatation and curettage		NAFPD	National Association of Family Planning Doctors
DHT	dihydrotestosterone			
DI	donor insemination		OHSS	ovarian hyperstimulation syndrome
DMPA	depot-medroxyprogesterone acetate		OPD	outpatients' department
dRVVT	dilute Russell viper venom time		PCC	postcoital contraception
DVT	deep vein thrombosis		PCOD	polycystic ovarian disease
ET	embryo transfer		PGF	prostaglandin F
FDA	Food and Drug Administration (US)		PID	pelvic inflammatory disease
FIGO	International Federation of Gynecology and Obstetrics		PMB	postmenopausal bleeding
			PMS	premenstrual syndrome
FMP	final menstrual period		POP	progestogen only pill
FPA	Family Planning Association		REM	rapid eye movement
FSH	follicle-stimulating hormone		RM	recurrent miscarriage
GIFT	gamete intra-fallopian transfer		SHBG	sex hormone binding globulin
GnRH	gonadotrophin releasing hormone		SLE	systemic lupus erythymatosis
GnRHag	gonadotrophin releasing hormone agonist		STOP	suction termination of pregnancy
			SUZI	subzonal sperm insertion
GSH	(symbol for) reduced glutathione		T3	triiodothyronine
GSI	genuine stress incontinence		T4	thyroxine
HCG	human chorionic gonadotrophin		TAH	total abdominal hysterectomy
HDL	high density lipoproteins		TOP	termination of pregnancy
HFEA	Human Fertilisation and Embryology Authority		TSH	thyroid stimulating hormone
			μg	microgram
HLA	human leucocyte antigen		UTI	urinary tract infection
HMG	human menopausal gonadotrophin		VAIN	vaginal intraepitheleal neoplasia
HPV	human papilloma virus		VDRL	Venereal Disease Reference Laboratory
HRT	hormone replacement therapy		VIN	vulval intraepithelial neoplasia
HSG	hysterosalpingography		WBC	white blood cell
IM	intramuscularly		WHO	World Health Organisation
iu	International Unit		ZIFT	zygote intra-fallopian transfer
IUCD	intrauterine contraceptive device			

1   A 17-year-old girl presents with primary amenorrhoea. Her karyotype is 45XO (Turner's syndrome). She is 1 m 47 cm (4 ft 10 in.) tall. She has a high arched palate, small lower jaw, short thick neck and a wide carrying angle of the arms. There is no breast development but some pubic and axillary hair growth. Which of the following statements are correct?

A) Her bone age would be appropriate for her age.   FALSE
B) She should be started on combined oestrogen/progesterone therapy to induce breast development.   FALSE
C) Ovulation could be induced with gonadotrophins when fertility is required.   FALSE
D) She has an increased risk of renal malformation.   TRUE
E) The incidence of Turner's syndrome per live birth is 1:2500.   TRUE

COMMENTS

Bone age, which is determined by the fusion of the epiphyseal cartilage in response to an increase in sex steroid, is delayed in girls with Turner's syndrome because sex steroid concentrations are reduced (Brook 1986).

Breast development is optimally achieved by mimicking the natural increase in oestrogen which occurs during puberty. Oestrogens are thus introduced in very small doses (2 µg daily), increasing to usual replacement doses over two years. Progestogens are added later to induce withdrawal bleeds.

In Turner's syndrome there are no remaining primordial follicles thus ovulation cannot be induced with gonadotrophins. About 50% of women with Turner's syndrome have abnormalities of renal development such as horseshoe kidney, renal aplasia or variation in the renal pelvis, ureters or blood vessels (Lippe et al. 1988).

REFERENCES

Brook, C.G.D. (1986) Turner's syndrome. *Arch Dis Child* **61**, 305-9

Lippe, B., Gefner, M.E., Dietrich, R.B. et al. (1988) Renal malformations in patients with Turner's syndrome: imaging in 141 patients. *Paediatrics* **82**, 852-6

2   In ectopic pregnancy:

A) The isthmus is the most common site for ectopic pregnancy in the fallopian tube.   FALSE

B) A high-quality vaginal sector probe will reliably detect a uterine gestational sac with a serum beta-HCG level between 1000 and 1500 iu/l.   FALSE

C) The Arias-Stella reaction in the endometrium is diagnostic of ectopic pregnancy.   FALSE

D) Continuing beta-HCG activity is found in 15% of ectopics after linear salpingostomy.   FALSE

E) Systemic methotrexate is not useful treatment for early cervical pregnancy.   FALSE

COMMENTS

Of all ectopic pregnancies, 97.7% occur in the fallopian tube; 1.3% are abdominal, 0.75% uterine and 0.15% ovarian. The commonest site for tubal pregnancies is the ampulla or infundibular portion of the tube followed by the isthmus and the interstitium (Breen 1970).

If the pregnancy test is positive and an ectopic pregnancy is suspected, a pelvic ultrasound assessment may be indicated. The sensitivity of a high-quality vaginal sector probe will usually detect a uterine sac with a serum beta-HCG level above 2000 iu/l (Nyberg et al. 1987).

Uterine curettage is occasionally useful. The presence of chorionic villi will confirm an intrauterine pregnancy but the Arias-Stella reaction is only present in 45-60% of ectopic pregnancies and therefore is not diagnostically sensitive or specific to ectopic pregnancy (Gordon 1980).

Laparoscopy is the investigation of choice for ectopic pregnancy which allows for the increasing frequency of conservative surgery using minimally invasive techniques.

Careful follow-up of patients treated by laparoscopic linear salpingotomy is required with twice weekly serum beta-HCG assays, as approximately 5% will have evidence of continuing trophoblastic activity (Vermesh et al. 1988).

Other conservative methods include expectant management in asymptomatic patients with falling levels of beta-HCG. Local injection of methotrexate and prostaglandin into the ectopic pregnancy with either laparoscopic or transvaginal ultrasound methods have also been described. Reports indicate that systemic methotrexate orally or parenterally has also been used and has been discussed as a useful treatment of early cervical pregnancy (Stovall et al. 1988).

REFERENCES

Breen, J.L. (1970) A 21-year survey of 654 ectopic pregnancies. *Am J Obstet Gynecol* **106**, 1004-19

Gordon, B.P. (1980) Frozen section examination of endometrial curettings: an aid to the rapid diagnosis of ectopic pregnancy. *Diagn Gynaecol Obstet* **2**, 77-80

Nyberg, D.A., Filly, R.A., Laing, F.C. *et al.* (1987) Ectopic pregnancy. Diagnosis by sonography correlated with quantitative HCG levels. *J Ultrasound Med* **6**, 145-50

Stovall, T.G., Ling, F.W., Smith, W.C. *et al.* (1988) Successful nonsurgical treatment of cervical pregnancy with methotrexate. *Fertil Steril* **50**, 672-4

Vermesh, M., Silva, P.D., Sauer, M.V. *et al.* (1988) Persistent tubal ectopic gestation; patterns of circulating beta-human chorionic gonadotrophin and progesterone, and management options. *Fertil Steril* **50**, 584-8

3   A 29-year-old nulliparous patient has had one mildly dyskaryotic smear, following two borderline smears over the previous 18 months. The management is as follows:

A) The smear should be repeated in three months.   FALSE
B) The patient should be referred for colposcopy.   TRUE
C) Human papilloma virus (HPV) viral typing should be performed on a sample from
the cervix.   FALSE ?
D) The patient's sexual partner should have penoscopy.   FALSE
E) The patient should be recommended to use condoms when having intercourse and
repeat the smear in six months.   FALSE

COMMENTS

The management of the low-grade smear remains controversial (Cooper *et al.* 1992). Repetition of the smear after an interval of three months would probably not seriously endanger the patient except that the uncertainty will do little to allay her fears.

Although referral for colposcopic opinion is a counsel of perfection it should be borne in mind that there is a considerable stress engendered by this procedure and the risk of overtreatment of a minor lesion is high (Soutter *et al.* 1986). However, in up to one third of mildly dyskaryotic smears, CIN III may be found, and there is a low but significant risk of an invasive lesion (Campion *et al.* 1986). The current recommendation for the management of these minor cytological changes is for referral to colposcopy, although trials are currently going on to assess the validity of this statement.

HPV typing is being aggressively pushed, by commercial concerns, in the USA, but the value of such information, which may also be of questionable accuracy, is limited. These tests are not recommended, as they simply produce more concern for the patient and little information for the clinician.

Penoscopy has been an interesting tool, but has proved to be of little or no clinical value. The use of condoms to 'protect' the cervix from noxious carcinogenic agents such as viruses is an attractive proposition, but has proved to be of little or no value. There is no current evidence to demonstrate that the spontaneous resolution of low-grade cytological abnormalities is improved by protection of the cervix by the use of condoms.

REFERENCES

Campion, M.J., McCance, D.J., Cuzick, J. *et al.* (1986) Progressive potential of mild cervical atypia: prospective cytological, colposcopic and virological study. *Lancet* 11, 237-40

Cooper, P., Kirby, A.J., Spiegelhalter, D.J. *et al.* (1992) Management of women with a cervical smear showing a mild degree of dyskaryosis: a review of policy. *Cytopathology* 3, 331-9

Soutter, W.P., Wisdom, S., Brough, A.K. *et al.* (1986) Should patients with mild atypia in a cervical smear be referred for colposcopy? *Br J Obstet Gynaecol* 93, 70-4

4 **A 32-year-old woman presents with lower abdominal pain. She gives a history of secondary infertility and recently has had *in vitro* fertilisation. Which of the following statements are correct?**

A) Her incidence of ectopic pregnancy is 3-4%.   FALSE
B) Serum beta-HCG level is diagnostic.   FALSE
C) The presence of an intrauterine pregnancy excludes an ectopic pregnancy.   FALSE
D) Positive serum HCG and ultrasound imaging produce a 99% positive predictive
   value.   TRUE
E) Laparoscopy is imperative.   FALSE

COMMENTS

Infertility and assisted conception are recogised risk factors for ectopic pregnancy (Dubuisson *et al.* 1991), with a significantly increased incidence.

Though quantitative beta-HCG radioimmunoassay remains the most sensitive endocrine test, it is not solely diagnostic.

The incidence of simultaneous intrauterine and extrauterine pregnancy increases with the advent of assisted conception techniques (Dimitry *et al.* 1990) and therefore statement (C), though generally applicable, does not hold true when ovarian superovulation is used.

In every woman in the reproductive age group with pelvic pain, particularly with a positive past history, ectopic pregnancy must be suspected and active effort must be made to confirm or rule out the diagnosis. The wider availability of serial beta-HCG measurement and vaginal sonography has made the early diagnosis more accurate but also avoids unnecessary laparoscopy and hospitalisation (Aleem *et al.* 1990).

REFERENCES

Aleem, F.A., DeFasio, M. and Gintautas, J. (1990) Endovaginal sonography for the early diagnosis of intrauterine and ectopic pregnancies. *Hum Reprod* **5**: 6, 755-8

Dimitry, E.S., Subak-Sharpe, R., Mills, M. *et al.* (1990) Nine cases of heterotopic pregnancies in four years of *in vitro* fertilisation. *Fertil Steril* **53**, 107-10

Dubuisson, J.B., Aubriot, F.X., Mathieu, L. *et al.* (1991) Risk factors for ectopic pregnancy in 556 pregnancies after *in vitro* fertilisation: implications for preventive management. *Fertil Steril* **56**: 4, 686-90

5   In ovarian cancer:

A) Advanced disease is seen in 45-55% of cases.   FALSE
B) Retroperitoneal nodal metastases are rare.   FALSE
C) Survival is related to the bulk of tumour present preoperatively.   TRUE
D) For all stages combined, the five-year survival is less than 30%.   TRUE
E) Autosomal dominant inheritance may occur.   TRUE

COMMENTS

It is well established by many studies that ovarian cancer presents with Stage III or IV disease in approximately 75% of cases. There is a significant degree of retroperitoneal lymph-node spread even in apparently early stage disease and this finding considerably decreases the prognosis (Di Re et al. 1989).

Stage	Lymph node metastases (%)
I	12.6
II	23.0
III	56.0
IV	64.7

It remains in doubt if major cyto-reductive surgery is beneficial (Hunter et al. 1992); however, the amount of disease present preoperatively is a clear independent indicator of prognosis (Hacker et al. 1983). For all stages the survival is less than 30%.

Ovarian cancer may be inherited. Site-specific ovarian cancer (Fraumeni et al. 1975) and breast/ovary (Lynch et al. 1978) families exhibit autosomal dominant inheritance with variable penetrance. Ovarian cancer occurring in Lynch Type II families shows multifactorial inheritance (Lynch et al. 1982).

REFERENCES

Di Re, F., Fontanelli, R., Raspagliesi, F. et al. (1989) 'Pelvic and para-aortic lymphadenectomy in cancer of the ovary' in E. Burghardt and J.M. Monaghan (Eds) Operative Treatment of Ovarian Cancer (Baillière's Clin Obstet Gynaecol) 3: 1, 131-42. London: Baillière Tindall

Fraumeni, J.F., Grundy, G.W., Creagan, E.T. et al. (1975) Six families prone to ovarian cancer. Cancer 36, 364-9

Hacker, N.F., Berek, J.S., Lagasse, L.D. et al. (1983) Primary cyto-reductive surgery for epithelial ovarian cancer. Obstet Gynecol 61, 413-20

Hunter, R.W., Neale, A.D.E., Soutter, W.P. (1992) Meta analysis of surgery in advanced ovarian carcinoma: is maximum cyto-reductive surgery an independent determinant of prognosis? Am J Obstet Gynecol 166, 504-11

Lynch, H.T., Harris, R.E., Guirgis, H.A. et al. (1978) Familial association of breast/ovarian carcinoma. Cancer 41, 1543-8

Lynch, H.T., Albano, W.A., Lynch, J.F. et al. (1982) Surveillance and management of patients at high genetic risk for ovarian cancer. Obstet Gynecol 59, 589-96

FURTHER READING

Burghardt, E. and Monaghan, J.M. (Eds) (1989) Operative Treatment of Ovarian Cancer (Baillière's Clin Obstet Gynaecol) 3: 1. London: Baillière Tindall

6 The antiprogesterone mifepristone (RU486):

A) Was licensed for use (in combination with a prostaglandin) for the termination of pregnancy in the UK in 1992.   FALSE
B) Is licensed for terminating pregnancies of up to 12 weeks' gestation.   FALSE
C) Also acts as an antiglucocortoid.   TRUE
D) Inhibits ovulation when administered daily in small doses.   TRUE
E) Is an effective post-coital contraceptive.   TRUE

COMMENTS

Mifepristone (RU486) was licensed for use in the UK in 1991 for termination of pregnancies up to nine weeks' gestation. Used beyond nine weeks the associated blood loss is too heavy for it to be an acceptable alternative to suction termination (blood loss is almost certainly related to the size of the placental site).

Mifepristone inhibits the binding of progesterone to its receptors and also inhibits glucocortoid receptor binding, although it does not appear to have any significant clinical effects at the doses currently in use. Progesterone is essential for the establishment of pregnancy as it ensures the orderly maturation of the endometrium, facilitating implantation.

Mifepristone given as a post-coital contraceptive has recently been shown to be as effective as – if not more effective than – the standard combination oestrogen/progestogen regime (Glasier *et al.* 1992; Webb *et al.* 1992). Given at a dose of 2 mg/day (Ledger *et al.* 1992), it inhibits ovulation. A number of pharmaceutical companies have antiprogesterone compounds which are said to be more potent than mifepristone. Over the next 10-20 years it is likely that their efficacy as contraceptives rather than as abortifacients will be investigated.

REFERENCES

Glasier, A., Thong, K.J., Dewar, M. *et al.* (1992) Randomised trial of mifepristone (RU486) and high dose estrogen-progestogen as an emergency contraceptive. *New Eng J Med* **327**, 1041-4

Webb, A.M.C., Russel, J. and Elstein, M. (1992) Comparison of the Yuzpe regimen, danazol and mifepristone in oral post-coital contraception. *BMJ* **305**, 927-31

Ledger, W.L., Sweeting, V.M., Hillier, H. *et al.* (1992) Inhibition of ovulation by low dose mifepristone (RU4860). *Hum Reprod* **7**, 945-50

7   A 35-year-old woman with menorrhagia is found to have uterine fibroids. An ultrasound scan suggests that the largest is 5 cm in diameter. The patient also has renal failure and is on peritoneal dialysis. She is nulliparous. Which of the following comments are correct?

A) She might benefit from endometrial ablation.	TRUE
B) Hysterectomy should be avoided.	TRUE
C) She could safely receive a gonadotrophin releasing hormone (GnRH) agonist alone on a long-term basis.	FALSE
D) The menstrual blood loss has a 70% chance of being decreased by a prostaglandin synthetase inhibitor.	FALSE
E) Fibroid shrinkage may be achieved with danazol.	FALSE

COMMENTS

Hysteroscopic techniques are ideal for treating this sort of patient. The chronically sick frequently wish to avoid major surgery and hysterectomy means that peritoneal dialysis will not be possible for at least three months and often longer. Sub-mucous fibroids up to 5 cm in diameter can be removed hysteroscopically although, if the uterine cavity is greater than about 11 cm or very distorted, the operation may be difficult or impossible. With a success rate of about 80% in reducing menstrual loss it is certainly worth a try. Endometrial ablation is likely to lead to infertility and must not be performed in those wanting further children.

If surgical treatment is contraindicated, then long-term agonist treatment may be used in combination with either HRT or medroxyprogesterone acetate given to relieve the postmenopausal side-effects (West *et al.* 1992). Unfortunately, bone density is difficult to assess in these patients who may have renal osteodystrophy. Danazol may produce temporary relief of symptoms but has no effect on the size of the fibroids.

REFERENCE

West, C.P., Lumsden, M.A., Hillier, H. *et al.* (1992) Potential role of medroxyprogesterone acetate as an adjunct to goserelin (Zoladex®) in the medical management of uterine fibroids. *Hum Reprod* **7**, 328-32

FURTHER READING

Fraser, I.S. (1992) 'Treatment of menorrhagia' in J.O. Drife and A.A. Calder (Eds) *Prostaglandins and the Uterus*, pp. 67-90. London: Springer-Verlag

8   A woman presenting with cyclical menorrhagia at the age of 46 years:

A) Has an 80% chance of having anovulatory cycles.   FALSE
B) Should be treated by dilatation and curettage.   FALSE
C) Is likely to be cured by hormone replacement therapy (HRT).   FALSE
D) Is likely to be cured by an oral progestogen.   FALSE
E) Is likely to require hysterectomy if medical treatment fails.   FALSE

COMMENTS

Women having regular menstrual cycles have an 80% chance of them being ovulatory. Although anovulation increases with age, it is usually associated with menstrual irregularity and even in the late 40s is less common than ovulation. Cyclical, oral progestogens are useful in those with irregular cycles since they improve the predictability of the menses, unpredictability being a major problem for many women even in the absence of excessive bleeding. However, there is no evidence that they have a significant effect on those with regular cycles (Cameron *et al.* 1990).

Hormone replacement therapy (HRT) contains only low doses of oestrogen and the woman's endogenous hormone production may swamp this, causing a worse problem. It is difficult to predict who will respond well but in some low-risk women the oral contraceptive pill may actually be more suitable. Also, the incidence of menorrhagia in those on HRT is similar to that in the population as a whole. Dilatation and curettage (D&C) is not a treatment for menorrhagia. It may be required for some with cyclical abnormality, although the endometrial samplers together with ultrasound and possibly hysteroscopy are likely to replace this operation in due course.

REFERENCE

Cameron, I.T., Haining, R., Lumsden, M.A. *et al.* (1990) The effects of mefanamic acid and norethisterone on measured menstrual blood loss. *Obstet Gynaecol* **76**, 85-8

FURTHER READING

Lumsden, M.A. (1992) 'Menstruation and menstrual abnormality' in R.W. Shaw, W.P. Soutter and S. Stanton (Eds) *Gynaecology*, pp. 189-204. Edinburgh: Churchill Livingstone

9   The combined oral contraceptive pill:

A) Is safe for women to use up to the menopause provided they are healthy non-smokers.   TRUE

B) Containing third-generation progestogens are more androgenic than pills containing norethisterone.   FALSE

C) May be associated with a slightly increased risk of early onset breast cancer in women who start to use it in their teens.   TRUE

D) Is associated with a reduction of almost 50% in the risk of both endometrial and ovarian cancer.   TRUE

E) A high-dose (50 μg oestrogen) preparation should be used by women taking the anticonvulsant sodium valproate.   FALSE

COMMENTS

With the reduction in the dose of oestrogen and the use of so-called third-generation progestogens the pill has become much safer. Recognising these changes, the Food and Drug Administration in the USA removed the upper age limit for use in healthy non-smokers. The new gestogens have a higher binding affinity for the progesterone receptor and lower affinity for the androgen receptor (Godsland et al. 1990). The relationship between long-term pill use and neoplasia was the subject of a WHO Scientific Group in 1991 which concluded that there was a minimal risk of early diagnosis of breast cancer (<3 years) in women who started the pill before the age of 25 (WHO 1992). The group also concluded that there was a highly significant protective effect against endometrial and ovarian cancer. Sodium valproate is an anticonvulsant which does not induce liver enzymes and therefore a higher dose of pill is not necessary (Szarewski and Guillebaud 1991).

REFERENCES

Godsland, I.F., Crook, D., Simpson, R. et al. (1990) The effects of different formulations of oral contraceptive agents on lipid and carbohydrate metabolism. New Eng J Med 323, 1375-81

Szarewski, A. and Guillebaud, J. (1991) Contraception. Current State of the Art. BMJ 302, 1224-6

WHO Scientific Group (1992) Oral Contraceptives and Neoplasia. WHO Technical Report Series 817. Geneva: World Health Organisation

10 Which of the following are associated with the development of vulval cancers?

A) Lichen sclerosis.	TRUE
B) Behçet's disease.	FALSE
C) Melanosis vulvae.	FALSE
D) Paget's disease.	TRUE
E) Vulval intraepithelial neoplasia (VIN) grade II.	TRUE

COMMENTS

The aetiology of carcinoma of the vulva is confusing, but there are several well-recognised conditions that appear to be premalignant. Approximately 4% of women with vulval lichen sclerosis develop invasive cancer (Meyrick Thomas *et al.* 1988), although lichen sclerosis and vulval intraepithelial neoplasia (VIN) may co-exist. The differentiation between the various grades of VIN is recommended by the Committee of the Nomenclature of the International Society for the Study of Vulvar Diseases (1989), but is probably clinically meaningless (Ferenczy 1991). All grades of VIN should be regarded with some suspicion, although the percentage progressing to invasive cancer is uncertain and may be as low as 4%. Paget's disease is uncommon but, as with Paget's disease of the breast, may become associated with an underlying apocrine tumour (25% of cases). Vulval Paget's may also be associated with tumours elsewhere. Behçet's disease is a benign ulcerative condition of the vulva, mouth and eye of unknown aetiology. Melanosis vulvae is a common pigmented lesion unrelated to malignant melanoma.

REFERENCES

Ferenczy, A. (1991) 'Intraepitheleal neoplasia of the vulva' in M. Coppleson, J.M. Monaghan, P. Morrow *et al.* (Eds) *Gynecologic Oncology* (2nd ed.), pp. 443-63. Edinburgh: Churchill Livingstone

International Society for the Study of Vulvar Diseases (1989) New nomenclature for vulvar disease. *Int J Gynaecol Pathol* **8**, 83

Meyrick Thomas, R.H., Ridley, C.M., McGibbon, D.H. *et al.* (1988) Lichen sclerosis and auto-immunity – a study of 350 women. *Br J Derm* **118**, 41-6

FURTHER READING

Soutter, W.P. (1992) 'Benign disease of the vulva and the vagina' in R.W. Shaw, W.P. Soutter and S. Stanton (Eds) *Gynaecology*, pp. 385-95. Edinburgh: Churchill Livingstone

11 Regarding male infertility:

A) The conception rate *in vivo* falls significantly at sperm concentrations of less than 5 million per ml.   **TRUE**

B) The presence of leucocytes in semen of an apparently healthy asymptomatic male has no prognostic significance.   **FALSE**

C) The fertilisation rates in *in vitro* fertilisation (IVF) are reduced if the initial sperm motility is less than 40%.   **TRUE**

D) *In vitro* fertilisation and tubal transfer (ET) are superior to gamete intra-fallopian transfer (GIFT) for treatment of male infertility.   **TRUE**

E) Subzonal sperm insertion (SUZI) for severe male infertility has resulted in an increased incidence of abnormal pregnancies.   **FALSE**

COMMENTS

The importance of sperm concentration is probably minimal if the other parameters are normal Jouannet and Feneaux (1987) have shown that the conception rate *in vivo* apparently only falls significantly at sperm concentrations of less than 5×10^6/ml.

Traditionally, an increase in the number or the presence of white blood cells (WBC) in semen has been taken to be one of the main clinical signs of genital tract infection. Barratt *et al.* (1992) have demonstrated that in patients with urethritis, the relationship between WBC and genital tract infection is contentious. Edwards *et al.* (1984) showed that oligospermia was not by any means the semen factor most deleterious to IVF outcome but that the presence of debris and leucocytes had a greater detrimental effect on fertilisation.

Mahadevan and Trounson (1984) reported reduced fertilisation rate if the sperm motility was 30%. Fertilisation failed with initial motility fewer than 20%. Barlow *et al.* (1991) have reported a correlation between fertilisation rate and post swim-up motility.

In vitro fertilisation and ET offer a better evaluation of the correlation between seminal parameters and fertility potential as expressed by fertilisation rate, which cannot be evaluated with GIFT (Oehninger *et al.* 1988). Tournaye *et al.* (1991) reported comparable ongoing pregnancy rate per transfer when comparing IVF and ZIFT (zygote intra-fallopian transfer).

The results of micromanipulation techniques have so far been disappointing. Partial zonal dissection may be useful for a small group of male factor patients but the problem of polyspermy remains. Subzonal insertion of sperm (SUZI) could result in fertilisation even with sperm motility of 2-10% with sperm densities ranging from 1.5-30 $\times 10^6$/ml. Of a total 369 oocytes (Fishel *et al.* 1990), 15% fertilised, with 0.5% polyspermy.

REFERENCES

Barlow, P., Delvigne, A., Van Drome, J. *et al.* (1991) Predictive value of classical and automated sperm analysis for *in vitro* fertilisation. *Hum Reprod* **6**, 1119-24

Barratt, C.L.R., Kessopoulou, E., Thompson, L.A. *et al.* (1992) The functional significance of leucocytes in human reproduction. *Reprod Med Rev* **1**, 115-29

Edwards, R.G., Fishel, S.B., Cohen, J. *et al.* (1984) Factors influencing the success of an *in vitro* fertilisation for alleviating human infertility. *J in Vitro Fert Embryo Transfer* **1**, 3-22

Fishel, S., Jackson, P., Antinori, S. *et al.* (1990) Subzonal insemination for the alleviation of infertility. *Fertil Steril* **54**, 828-35

Jouannet, P. and Feneaux, D. (1987) Sperm analysis. *Ann Biol Clin* **45**, 335-41

Mahadevan, M.M. and Trounson, A.D. (1984) The influence of seminal characteristics on the success rate of human *in vitro* fertilization. *Fertil Steril* **42**, 400-5

Oehninger, S., Acosta, A.A., Krugger, T. *et al.* (1988) Failure of fertilization in *in vitro* fertilization; the occult male factor. *J in Vitro Fert Embryo Transfer* **5**, 181

Tournaye, H., Camus, M., Khan, I. *et al.* (1991) *In vitro* fertilisation, gamete or zygote intrafallopian transfer for the treatment of male infertility. *Hum Reprod* **6**, 263-6

12 Premenstrual symptoms:

A)	Usually occur during GnRH analogue therapy.	FALSE
B)	Are experienced by 95% of women.	TRUE
C)	Frequently occur during cyclical hormone replacement therapy.	TRUE
D)	Can be diagnosed by assessing an endocrine profile.	FALSE
E)	Are reliably treated by high-dose progesterone.	FALSE

COMMENTS

GnRH agonist analogues have been very successful in treating premenstrual syndrome. However, whenever GnRH analogues are used for any indication they do cause symptoms of the menopause due to the markedly reduced oestrogen production. The value of therapy is limited by the risks of osteoporosis and cardiovascular disease. Premenstrual symptoms do occur in 95% of women. In the majority these are mild and can be considered normal physiological events of the hormone cycle. When the symptoms are severe enough to interfere with a woman's normal functioning then it can be considered as premenstrual syndrome (PMS). The prevalence of true PMS has never been accurately assessed but is far less than 95% (O'Brien 1992).

When unopposed oestrogen replacement is given to women, premenstrual symptoms virtually never occur. However, in women with an intact uterus it is necessary to give cyclical progestogen to protect the endometrium from hyperplasia and endometrial cancer. The cyclical progestogen is associated with symptomatic side-effects which are similar to those of PMS. They can occasionally be sufficiently distressing that the woman discontinues the HRT or, perhaps worse, omits the progestogen.

No endocrine test is of value in diagnosing PMS. Some research workers have suggested that a low level of sex hormone binding globulin can pinpoint these patients. There are unfortunately no objective tests for PMS and the diagnosis must be based on prospectively administered symptom rating charts. There have been many claims that 'pure' progesterone is effective in the management of PMS but virtually every properly controlled study contradicts this (Freeman *et al.* 1990).

REFERENCES

Freeman, E., Rickells, K., Sondheimer, S.J. *et al.* (1990) Ineffectiveness of progesterone suppository treatment for premenstrual tension. *JAMA* **264**, 349-53

O'Brien, P.M.S. (1992) 'Premenstrual syndrome' in R.W. Shaw, W.P. Soutter and S. Stanton (Eds) *Gynaecology,* pp. 325-39. Edinburgh: Churchill Livingstone

13 In pelvic tuberculosis:

A)	In over 80% of cases, the primary focus is in the lungs.	TRUE
B)	Cervical lesions can sometimes be mistaken for cervical carcinoma.	TRUE
C)	Curettage is best done in the first half of the menstrual cycle.	FALSE
D)	Rifampicin may reduce the effectiveness of the oral contraceptive.	TRUE
E)	Optic neuritis is associated with ethambutol treatment.	TRUE

COMMENTS

The natural history of pelvic tuberculosis has been outlined by Barnes (1955). In most cases tuberculosis infection of the female genital tract is secondary to a primary focus elsewhere in the body. In over 80% of cases the primary focus is in the lungs. In about 90% of Sutherland's series (Sutherland 1975), a history of an extragenital lesion or evidence of healed or active pulmonary tuberculosis, calcified abdominal glands or urinary tuberculosis was found.

The lesion when on the cervix either resembles an ulcer or is proliferative and could be mistaken for carcinoma (Novak and Woodruff 1974).

The results of culture and/or guinea pig inoculation have a higher success rate premenstrually, and therefore material should be obtained in the second half of the cycle.

Rifampicin causes induction of microsomal hepatic enzymes and therefore reduces the effectiveness of warfarin, phenytoin, sulphonylureas, oestrogen oral contraceptives and corticosteroids. Ethambutol may produce a unique type of visual impairment which is generally reversible and appears to be due to optic neuritis and to be related to dose and duration of treatment (Citron and Thomas 1986). It is recommended that, before commencing ethambutol, all patients have a full opthalmic examination involving acuity, colour vision, perimetry and opthalmoscopy and that patients should be informed of the importance of reporting any changes in vision.

REFERENCES

Barnes, T. (1955) The natural history of pelvic tuberculosis. *J Obstet Br Emp* **62**, 162-75

Citron, K.M. and Thomas, G.O. (1986) Ocular toxicity from ethambutol. *Thorax* **41**, 737-9

Novak, E.R. and Woodruff, J.D. (1974) *Gynaecologic and Obstetric Pathology*, pp. 308-9. London: W.B. Saunders

Sutherland, A.M. (1975) Gynaecological tuberculosis, past, present and future. *Arch Gynecol* **218**, 261-8

14 **With regard to Tibolone, which may be used for hormone replacement therapy, which of the following statements are correct?**

A) It is not active when given orally.	FALSE
B) It causes endometrial stimulation in 10% of women.	TRUE
C) It is ineffective in conserving bone mass.	FALSE
D) It has no effect on gonadotrophins.	FALSE
E) Progesterone addition is not required.	TRUE

COMMENTS

Tibolone is an orally active preparation which is unique in having simultaneous oestrogenic, progestogenic and androgenic properties (Wardle and Padwick 1992). When given continuously it has been shown to alleviate oestrogen deficiency symptoms. Although only slight, endometrial proliferation may occur in 10% of women, and this may lead to troublesome breakthrough bleeding (Genazzani *et al.* 1991). However, progestogens are not required in the absence of such bleeding. In placebo-controlled studies, tibolone has been shown to prevent postmenopausal bone loss, and may even be effective in preventing further bone loss in women with established osteoporosis (Lindsay *et al.* 1980).

Tibolone has been shown to suppress FSH and LH levels in postmenopausal women, and may suppress ovulation in fertile women (Benedek-Jaszmann 1991).

REFERENCES

Benedek-Jaszmann, L.J. (1991) Long term placebo-controlled efficacy and safety study of ORG OD 14 in climacteric women. *Maturitas* **1 (Suppl)**, 25-33

Genazzani, A.R., Benedek-Jaszmann, L.J. and Hart, D.M. (1991) ORG OD 14 and the endometrium. *Maturitas* **13**, 243-51

Lindsay, R., Hart, D.M. and Krasewski, A. (1980) A prospective double blind trial of synthetic steroid (Org 15) for preventing postmenopausal osteoporosis. *BMJ* **280**, 1207-9

Wardle, P.G. and Padwick, M.L. (1992) Hormone replacement therapy. *Hospital Update* **June**, 443-54

15 Regarding adenocarcinoma-in-situ of the cervix:

A) The average age of women at diagnosis of adenocarcinoma-in-situ of the cervix is 50 years.   FALSE

B) Few cases of adenocarcinoma-in-situ of the cervix are detected as a result of an abnormal cytology report.   FALSE

C) CIN is seen together with adenocarcinoma of the cervix in 50% of cases.   TRUE

D) The depth of the cone biopsy should include at least 20 mm of the endocervical canal.   FALSE

E) If hysterectomy is performed for adenocarcinoma-in-situ of the cervix, ovarian conservation should take place.   TRUE

COMMENTS

The average age at diagnosis of adenocarcinoma-in-situ of the cervix is between 25 and 40 years in most series, which is ten years less than the median age for invasive adenocarcinoma (Luesley et al. 1987).

Routine cervical cytology is the most common method by which women with adenocarcinoma-in-situ are diagnosed. Cytologic criteria have been established and include exfoliated sheets of cells with palisading and pseudostratification of nuclei.

Up to 50% of patients with adenocarcinoma-in-situ of the cervix will also have squamous cervical intraepithelial neoplasia (CIN) (Ayer et al. 1987).

Colposcopy and punch biopsy do not provide sufficient information or tissue to exclude invasive adenocarcinoma. Cone biopsy is the method by which the histological diagnosis of adenocarcinoma-in-situ can be made.

The ectocervical margins are best determined by colposcopy but the depth of the cone should include at least 25 mm of the endocervical canal (Hopkins et al. 1988).

Follow-up and cytologic assessment may be complicated and most authors recommend hysterectomy as the treatment of choice. However, evidence that these lesions are multifocal is limited. Ostor et al. (1984) found only three out of 20 patients with multifocal disease and no patient had residual disease in the hysterectomy specimen where cone biopsy had free margins. Series such as these are reassuring in those individualised cases where fertility is important and conservative management is undertaken. Close follow-up is mandatory in these situations.

In the young patient where hysterectomy is undertaken there is no contraindication to ovarian conservation (Bertrand et al. 1987).

REFERENCES

Ayer, B., Pacey, F., Greenberg, M. et al. (1987) The cytologic diagnosis of adenocarcinoma-in-situ of the cervix uteri and related lesions. 1: Adenocarcinoma in situ. Acta Cytol **31**, 397-41

Bertrand, M., Lickrish, G.M. and Colgan, T.J. (1987) The anatomic distribution of cervical adenocarcinoma-in-situ: implications for treatment. Am J Obstet Gynecol **157**, 21-5

Hopkins, M.P., Roberts, J.A. and Schmidt, R.W. (1988) Cervical adenocarcinoma-in-situ. Obstet Gynecol **71**, 842-4

Luesley, D.M., Jordan, J.A., Woodman, C.B.J. et al. (1987) A retrospective review of adenocarcinoma-in-situ and glandular atypia of the uterine cervix. Br J Obstet Gynaecol **94**, 699-703

Ostor, A.G., Pagano, R., Davoren, R.A.M. et al. (1984) Adenocarcinoma-in- situ of the cervix. Int J Gynecol Pathol **3**, 179-90

16 Coronary heart disease in women:

A) Is the major single cause of death in Western Europe. — TRUE
B) Is increased in users of the oral contraceptive pill. — FALSE
C) The differential increase in death rates after the menopause (compared to men) is clearly due to loss of endogenous oestrogen. — FALSE
D) Oestrogen replacement therapy reduces risk by 50%. — ~~TRUE~~ *False*
E) Oestrogen replacement therapy (combined with a progestogen to protect from endometrial carcinoma) may reduce risk by 50%. — ~~TRUE~~ *False*

with study

COMMENTS

Cardiovascular disease is the leading cause of death in women after the menopause in most developed countries – far exceeding the numbers caused by cancer (Sitruik-Ware 1991). This is the case even in countries where overall coronary mortality has been declining (Uemura and Pisa 1988). For example, twice as many women die each year from heart disease and stroke in the USA than do those from all cancers combined. Coronary heart disease alone accounts for more than 36% of all deaths in women (Bush and Miller 1987).

A review of the nine observational studies of heart disease in former users of the oral contraceptive pill reveals no evidence of increased risk (Barrett-Connor and Bush 1991).

The sex differential in death rates from coronary heart disease does diminish with age (Vessey and Hunt 1988) but this may be due to a reduction in the rates of increase in men rather than an increase in women (Godsland et al. 1987).

Quantitative evaluation of published studies (by meta analysis) suggests oestrogen use is associated with a 50% reduction of cardiovascular occurrence. Qualitative evaluation suggests this association is causal as it fits five of the six epidemiological criteria for causality (consistency of association, proper time sequence, strength of association, change in risk with change of exposure, and biological plausibility) (Bush 1991). It is therefore true to say that oestrogen replacement therapy reduces risk of coronary heart disease by 50%.

Although there is little evidence of cardiovascular risk in menopausal women on oestrogen–progestogen compounds (Bush 1991), and adverse lipid effects of progestogens might imply a reduction in the protective effect of oestrogen (Ross et al. 1990), a review of the three studies which have assessed risk suggest this is not the case (Samsioe 1991). The largest and most recent of these revealed a reduction in coronary risk of 50% (Persson et al. 1990). It is therefore true to say that oestrogen replacement therapy combined with progestogen may reduce the risk of coronary heart disease by 50%.

REFERENCES

Barrett-Connor, E. and Bush, T.L. (1991) Estrogen and coronary heart disease in women. *J Am Med Assoc* **265**: 14, 1861-7

Bush, T.L. (1991) Extraskeletal effects of estrogen and the prevention of atherosclerosis. *Osteoporosis Int* **2**, 5-11

Bush, T.L. and Miller, V. (1987) 'Effects of pharmacologic agents used during menopause: impact on lipids and lipoproteins' in D. Mishell (Ed.) *Menopause, Physiology and Pharmacology*, pp. 187-208. Chicago: Year Book Medical Publications

Godsland, I.F., Wynn, V., Crook, D. et al. (1987) Sex, plasma lipoproteins, and atherosclerosis: prevailing assumptions and outstanding questions. *Am J Med* **114**, 1467

Persson, I., Falkeborn, M. and Lithell, H. (1990) 'The effect on myocardial infarction risk of estrogens and estrogen–progestin combinations'. Proceedings of the 6th International Congress on the Menopause, Bangkok. Abst. 219, p. 223

Ross, R.K., Pike, M.C., Mack, T.M. et al. (1990) 'Oestrogen replacement therapy and cardiovascular disease' in J.O. Drife and J.W.W. Studd (Eds) *HRT and Osteoporosis*, pp. 217-18. London: Springer-Verlag

Samsioe, G. (1991) 'Cardiovascular disease and lipid metabolism: the influence of HRT' in W.H. Utian, B.L. Riggs and G. Samsioe (Eds) *Long-term HRT*, p. 22. Carnforth: Parthenon Publishing

Sitruik-Ware, R. (1991) 'Do estrogens protect against cardiovascular disease? ' in R. Sitruik-Ware and W.H. Utian (Eds) *The Menopause and Hormone Replacement Therapy*, p. 161. New York: Marcel Dekker

Uemura, K. and Pisa, Z. (1988) Recent trends in cardiovascular disease mortality in 27 industrialised countries. *World Health Stat Q* **38**, 142-62

Vessey, M. and Hunt, K. (1988) 'The menopause, hormone replacement therapy and cardiovascular disease: epidemiological aspects' in J.W.W. Studd, and M.I. Whitehead (Eds) *The Menopause*, p. 190. Oxford: Blackwell Scientific

17 The use of LHRH analogues for uterine fibromyomata:

A) Is usually limited to six months.	TRUE
B) Is sometimes associated with acute haemorrhage.	TRUE
C) May be associated with severe pain in the shrinking fibroids.	TRUE
D) The use of analogue with a progestogen may achieve fibroid shrinkage without loss of bone mass.	TRUE
E) Tamoxifen alters the size of uterine fibroids.	FALSE

COMMENTS

Hackenburg and colleagues (1992) report: 'in most cases it seems to be possible to estimate the individual response to GnRH application after the first injection so that it is possible to stop therapy in non-responding patients'. After three months, 15% of 27 fibroids showed a greater than 50% reduction in volume and one complete remission was achieved. At present treatment is usually limited to six months and there is no evidence of further reduction in size if treatment is continued for longer than this. The reduction in size does not persist after completion of treatment.

Submucous myomas treated with GnRH have reported to result in profuse haemorrhage (Thorpe and Katz 1991).

REFERENCES

Hackenburg, R. *et al.* (1992) *Eur J Obstet Gynecol Reprod Biol* **45**: 2, 125-9

Thorpe, J.M. and Katz, V.L. (1991) Submucous myomas treated with gonadotrophin releasing hormone agonist and resulting in vaginal haemorrhage: a case report. *J Reprod Med* **36**: 8, 625-6

FURTHER READING

Chipato, T., Healy, D.L., Vollenhoven, B. *et al.* (1991) Pelvic pain complicating LHRH analogue treatment of fibroids. *Aust NZ J Obstet Gynaecol* **31**: 4, 383-4

Maheux, R., Lemay, A., Blanchet, P. *et al.* (1991) Maintained reduction of uterine leiomyoma following addition of hormonal replacement therapy to monthly luteinizing hormone releasing hormone agonist implant: a pilot study. *Hum Reprod* **6**: 4, 500-5

Lumsden, M.A., West, C.P. and Baird, D.T. (1989) Tamoxifen prolongs luteal phase in premenopausal women but has no effect on the size of the uterine fibroids. *J Clin Endocrinol* **31**: 3 335-43

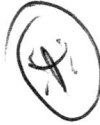

18 **The following statements apply to carcinoma of the cervix:**

A) Adeno, squamous and tumours of mixed histological type all arise from transition zone epithelium.   TRUE

B) Ninety per cent are pure squamous cell tumours.   FALSE

C) Mixed adenosquamous tumours are associated with poorer survival rates than pure adenocarcinomas.   TRUE

D) The presence of vascular space permeation is a prognostic indicator independent of lymph node status.   TRUE

E) The risk of lymph node metastases in women with microinvasive disease increases from 0.5% to 3% when comparing lesions with a depth penetration <3 mm to those of 3–5 mm.   FALSE

COMMENTS

Histogenically, the majority of cervical malignancies are believed to arise from the reserve stem cell of the transition zone epithelium. Divergent differentiation towards squamous, glandular or a mixed pattern is therefore possible (Teshima *et al.* 1985).

Only about 70% of cervical carcinomas are pure squamous lesions. The routine use of mucin stains has resulted in 20–30% of tumours previously regarded as squamous being reclassified as poorly differentiated adenocarcinomas or as mixed adenosquamous tumours (Buckley *et al.* 1988).

Women with adenosquamous tumours have significantly higher local recurrence rates and poorer survival when compared to simple adenocarcinomas and non-mucin producing squamous tumours (Bethwaite *et al.* 1982).

The presence of vascular space permeation by cervical tumours is known to be associated with a poor clinical outlook and may be used as an independent prognostic indicator (Buckley *et al.* 1988).

The risk of lymph node metastases increases significantly to 8% when the depth of penetration is between 3 and 5 mm (Maiman *et al.* 1988).

REFERENCES

Bethwaite, P., Yeong, M.L., Holloway, L. *et al.* (1982) The prognosis of adenosquamous carcinomas of the uterine cervix. *Br J Obstet Gynaecol* **99**, 745-50

Buckley, C., Beards, C. and Fox, H. (1988) Pathological prognostic indicators in cervical cancer with particular reference to patients under the age of 40 years. *Br J Obstet Gynaecol* **95**, 47-56

Maiman, M., Fruchter, R., Di Maio, T. *et al.* (1988) Superficially invasive squamous cell carcinoma of the cervix. *Obstet Gynecol* **72**, 399-403

Teshima, S., Shimosato, Y., Kishi, K. *et al.* (1985) Early stage adenocarcinoma of the uterine cervix: histopathologic analysis with consideration of histogenesis. *Cancer* **56**, 167-72

19 Regarding contraception for the woman over 35:

A) Because of a considerably increased risk of breast cancer, the use of the combined oral contraceptive (COC) should be discouraged.   FALSE

B) Healthy women over 35 years of age, without coronary artery disease risk factors, can use low-dose oral contraception with confidence.   TRUE

C) The use of COC results in a significant decrease in the occurrence of functional ovarian cysts.   TRUE

D) Progestin-releasing intrauterine devices lead to an increased incidence of heavy bleeding.   FALSE

E) The ratio of ectopic pregnancy to total pregnancies conceived is higher with progestin-only IUDs, compared with that of copper-containing IUDs.   TRUE

COMMENTS

The influence of oral contraceptives on breast-cancer incidence continues to be discussed. A meta analysis of 27 published studies did not find any significant increase in the incidence of breast cancer in oral pill users. A slight increase in the occurrence rate of younger women with prolonged use of oral contraceptives was found (Rushton and Jones 1992; Wingo *et al.* 1991).

Cardiovascular disease (CVD) incidence increases with age in women. The principal risk factor is cigarette smoking. The other risk factors for developing CVD are hypertension, diabetes mellitus, hyperlipidaemia, family history of early onset of CVD, and obesity. Non-smokers over the age of 35 who use oral contraceptives have only a slight increase in CVD incidence compared with non-oral contraceptive users. The incidence has been estimated to be only one or two cases per 100 000 women (Thorogood *et al.* 1991).

The incidence of functional ovarian cysts decreases in relationship to the formulation of the oral contraception, the effect being more marked with monophasic formulations and containing oestrogens >35 μg when compared with the use of the multiphasic pill (Lanes *et al.* 1992).

A major problem with IUDs has been the increased incidence of heavy bleeding or cramping associated with their use. Progestin-releasing IUDs have been found to reduce the amount of uterine bleeding associated with menstruation (Milsom *et al.* 1991). Ectopic pregnancy is another concern with IUD use. The chance of occurrence of an ectopic pregnancy is slightly higher with progestin-only IUDs. It is therefore important to rule out an ectopic pregnancy if the woman complains of lower quadrant pain with a positive pregnancy test (Sivin 1991).

REFERENCES

Lanes, S.F., Birman, B., Walker, A.M. *et al.* (1992) Oral contraceptive types and functional ovarian cysts. *Am J Obstet Gynecol* **166**, 956-61

Milsom, I., Andersson, K., Andersch, B. *et al.* (1991) A comparison of flurbiprofen, tranexamic acid and a levonorgestrel-releasing intrauterine contraceptive device in the treatment of idiopathic menorrhagia. *Am J Obstet Gynecol* **164**, 3, 879-83

Rushton, L. and Jones, D.R. (1992) Oral contraceptive use and breast cancer risk: a meta-analysis of variations with age at diagnosis, parity and total duration of oral contraceptive use. *Br J Obstet Gynaecol* **99**, 230-46

Sivin, I. (1991) Dose and age dependent ectopic pregnancy risks associated with intrauterine conception. *Obstet Gynecol* **78**, 291-8

Thorogood, M., Mann, J., Murphy, M. *et al.* (1991) Is oral contraceptive use still associated with an increased risk of fatal myocardial infarction? Report of a case control study. *Br J Obstet Gynaecol* **98**, 1245-53

Wingo, P.A., Lee, N.C., Ory, H.W. *et al.* (1991) Age specific differences in the relationship between oral contraceptive use and breast cancer. *Obstet Gynecol* **78**, 161-70

20 A 52-year-old, postmenopausal married woman presents to her gynaecologist with severe vulvar discomfort, irritation and occasional vulvar pain. Clinical examination reveals cracked epithelium, with white patches of thickened skin. The management is as follows:

A) Take vulvar swabs for bacteriology and prescribe a broad spectrum antibiotic.   FALSE
B) Refer for vulvoscopy and biopsy under local anaesthetic.   TRUE
C) Prescribe short-term dilute hydrocortisone cream and review.   FALSE
D) Immediate biopsy of representative white patches under local anaesthetic.   TRUE
E) Prescribe testosterone proprionate cream and review in three months.   FALSE

COMMENTS

It is important to eliminate local infection and infestation with agents such as *Candida*. However, simple swabs are rarely helpful due to contamination from skin flora and perineal soiling with bacteria from the anus. Candidiasis is often deeply seated and is best identified on scrapings from the vulva. Broad spectrum antibiotics are singularly unhelpful and may alter the delicate milieu to an even greater extent, generating further difficulties. The use of oestrogen creams also appears unhelpful in the majority of patients. If there is a vulvar clinic available in the district and the gynaecologist feels that a better opinion can be given, then referral to such a clinic will be helpful in the management of these problems.

Short-term therapy with hydrocortisone is commonly used but appears to maximise the damage from steroids and fails to achieve long-term benefits. Testosterone creams have been widely used for empirical treatment of vulvar irritation, but studies have shown an equivalent effect from simple placebos. Recent data suggest that for lichen sclerosis the use of long-term (three months) clobetasol 0.05% (Dermovate®) achieves an excellent response for many patients.

However, prior biopsy is mandatory and most gynaecologists would be comfortable and skilled enough to carry out the simple procedures in the outpatients under local anaesthesia. The addition of the colposcope provides illumination and magnification to facilitate identification of the appropriate site of such biopsies. Once an histological opinion has been received, decisions can be made about further treatment. Currently, with the wide availability of colposcopic outpatient facilities, it is very simple to biopsy lesions in the clinic. It is only the occasional patient who will require a general anaesthetic.

SUGGESTED READING

Singer, A., Monaghan, J.M. and Richart, R. (Eds) (1994) *Lower Genital Tract Precancer: Colposcopy, Pathology and Treatment.* Oxford: Blackwell Scientific

21 Approaching the time of menopause, women:

A) Can remain fertile even with a raised FSH level. — TRUE
B) Should stop the combined oral contraceptive pill. — FALSE
C) If taking a progestogen-only pill, may become amenorrhoeic. — TRUE
D) May change contraception from the combined pill to HRT. — FALSE
E) With an IUCD in situ can expect irregular vaginal bleeding. — FALSE

COMMENTS

At the menopause, serum oestrogen levels fall and pituitary gonadotrophin levels rise. However, oestrogen levels can remain high after the final period, and FSH and LH levels can be raised for a year or more before the last period. FSH levels above 15 iu/l on two occasions separated by at least three months usually indicate no further need for contraception. Pregnancy has, however, been reported in these circumstances (Metcalf *et al.* 1982).

There is no upper age limit for use of the newer combined oral contraceptives (COCs) in normotensive, non-smoking women (Fortney 1990). Preference should be given to preparations containing a 'third generation' progestogen such as norgestimate, gestodene or desogestrel (Parsons 1993).

Some women taking the progestogen-only pill (POP) become amenorrhoeic. The POP does not suppress the rise in FSH at the menopause, and this should be measured in amenorrhoeic women over the age of 45 (Guillebaud 1992).

Women who take HRT before their final period remain fertile, so need non-hormonal methods of contraception. The IUCD may aggravate the menorrhagia that many women experience premenopausally. However, the IUCD does not cause intermenstrual bleeding, and under these circumstances endometrial biopsy should be considered.

REFERENCES

Fortney, J.A. (1990) Oral contraceptives for older women. *IPPF Med Bull* **24**, 3-4

Guillebaud, J. (1992) Contraception for women over 35 years of age. *Br J Fam Plann* **17**, 15-18

Metcalf, M.G., Donald, R.A. and Livesey, J.H. (1982) Pituitary-ovarian function before, during and after the menopause: a longitudinal study. *Clin Endocrinol* **17**, 5, 489-94

Parsons, T. (1993) HRT and contraception. *Br J Sex Med* **20**, 22-3

22 In development of human sexual physical identity, which of the following statements are true?

A) The human embryo will develop into a phenotypic female in the absence of any other stimuli. TRUE

B) Anti-Müllerian factor initiates the development of the testes and subsequent inhibition of Müllerian duct development. FALSE

C) In a case of female congenital adrenal hyperplasia the infant will have both Müllerian and wolffian duct development. FALSE

D) In a case of testicular feminisation due to 5-alpha reductase deficiency, the individual will have an absent prostate but normal seminal vesicles. TRUE

E) H-Y antigen is responsible for the migration of germ cells from the yolk sac into the developing testes. FALSE

COMMENTS

Normal development of sex begins at fertilisation with the chromosomal sex being determined by the type and number of sex chromosomes present in the conceptus. Regardless of chromosomal sex the early embryo is sexually bipotent and can develop either (or both) sets of sexual organs. H-Y antigen secreted at the sixth week initiates development of the testes but not germ-cell migration into it. If H-Y antigen is not forthcoming the gonadal ridge will differentiate into ovaries at the 13th week; indeed the neuter state of the human is female and suppression of Müllerian development requires the presence of a specific inhibitor, anti-Müllerian factor (AMF). AMF is a glycoprotein produced by Sertoli cells, and it is not related to testosterone or H-Y antigen. Its action is confined locally not systemically, illustrated by the findings of wolffian structures which are confined to the ipsilateral side of the testes in cases of TRUE hermaphrodism. Wolffian duct development requires the presence of testosterone; however, complete virilisation of the cloaca (which includes prostate development) requires dihydrotestosterone (DHT) and hence the presence of the 5-alpha reductase enzymes which convert testosterone to DHT. Congenital adrenal hyperplasia (CAH) does not cause wolffian development as the insult happens too late in fetal life to stimulate its development.

APPROPRIATE READING

Ohno, S., Nagai, Y., Ciccarese, S. *et al.* (1979) Testis organising H-Y antigen and the primary sex determining mechanism in mammals. *Recent Prog Hormone Res* **35**, 449-70

Peterson, R.E., Imperato-McGinley, J., Gautier, T. *et al.* (1977) Male pseudo hermaphroditism due to steroid 5-alpha reductase deficiency. *Am J Med* **62**, 170-9

Shearman, R.P. (1985) 'Intersexuality' in *Clinical Reproductive Endocrinology*, pp. 346-97. Edinburgh: Churchill Livingstone

Wilson, J.D., Griffin, J.E., George, F.W. *et al.* (1981) The role of gonadal steroids in sexual differentiation. *Recent Prog Hormone Res* **37**, 1-33

23 Conservative management of ectopic pregnancy by intratubal injection of methotrexate:

A) Is contraindicated in the presence of tubal rupture. TRUE

B) Should be limited to cases with a tubal diameter of 3–4 cm. TRUE

C) Is particularly effective when ultrasound examination demonstrates fetal cardiac activity. FALSE

D) Should be followed by serial measurement of serum progesterone until values fall to the non-pregnant range. FALSE

E) Is safe provided that citrovorum factor is administered concurrently. FALSE

COMMENTS

Systemic methotrexate was used initially to treat ectopic pregnancy (Tanaka *et al.* 1982) and later combined with citrovorum rescue (folinic acid) in an attempt to limit toxicity. Intratubal injection of methotrexate appears to be as effective, however, and as the total dosage is greatly reduced systemic toxicity is unlikely (Pansky *et al.* 1989). Conservative treatment methods appear more likely to fail in the presence of high titres of serum HCG or fetal cardiac activity seen on ultrasound. Most workers limit injection methods to small unruptured ectopics. Other strategies such as laparoscopic linear salpingostomy may, however, allow a conservative approach to be adopted in the majority of women including those with tubal rupture (Pouly *et al.* 1986). Conservative management may fail in 5–10% of cases and therefore it is important to confirm that viable trophoblast has been effectively eradicated by performing serial HCG assays to identify cases which may require additional therapy.

REFERENCES

Pansky, M., Bukovsky, I., Golan, A. *et al.* (1989) Local methotrexate injection: a non-surgical treatment of ectopic pregnancy. *Am J Obstet Gynecol* **161**, 393-6

Pouly, J.L., Mahnes, H., Mage, G. *et al.* (1986) Conservative laparoscopic treatment of 321 ectopic pregnancies. *Fertil Steril* **46**, 1093-7

Tanaka, T., Hayashi, H., Kutsuzawa, T. *et al.* (1982) Treatment of interstitial ectopic pregnancy with methotrexate: report of a successful case. *Fertil Steril* **37**, 851-2

24 **In the treatment of genuine stress incontinence (GSI):**

A) Physiotherapy will improve symptoms in about 20% of patients.   FALSE
B) Patients with co-existent detrusor instability should not undergo surgical treatment.   FALSE
C) Preoperative urethral pressure profilometry can predict the success of surgical treatment.   TRUE
D) Colposuspension is the commonest surgical treatment employed by gynaecologists in the UK.   FALSE
E) At colposuspension good elevation of the bladder neck is a critical factor in determining success.   FALSE

COMMENTS

Whilst physiotherapy will only cure about 20% of patients with GSI, cure and improvement rates are consistently around 70% especially with the use of vaginal cones (Wilson *et al.* 1987; Bridges *et al.* 1988). As no consistent predictive factors can be found many urogynaecologists feel a trial of physiotherapy is warranted before any surgical procedure. Although the success of surgical treatment is poorer in the presence of high-pressure detrusor instability, low-pressure detrusor instability does not seem to adversely affect success rates (Lockhart *et al.* 1993). Coexistent detrusor instability should not therefore be considered an absolute contraindication to bladder neck surgery, especially if it is of 'low pressure' type (<25 cm H_2O), and especially where conservative treatment of both conditions has failed.

Patients with a maximal urethral closure pressure of <20 cm H_2O are three times more likely to have an unsatisfactory outcome to their colposuspension (Sand *et al.* 1987). This is one of the reasons why urodynamic investigations are recommended before surgical treatment, especially after failed previous surgery.

Despite widespread evidence that suprapubic surgery has a much greater cure rate overall than colporrhaphy, a survey of gynaecologists in the UK showed that anterior colporrhaphy was four times more commonly performed than colposuspension as a treatment of GSI (Hilton 1988).

While elevation of the bladder neck is important in colposuspension, it appears to be the proximity of it to the back of the symphysis that determines success or failure. The enhancement of pressure transmission ratios to greater than 100% in the proximal urethra following successful colposuspension probably reflects compression of the proximal urethra against the symphysis during coughing, straining, etc.

REFERENCES

Bridges, N. *et al.* (1988) A prospective trial comparing interferential therapy and treatment using cones in patients with symptoms of stress incontinence. *Neurourol Urodyn* **7**, 259-61

Hilton, P. (1988) Bladder drainage. A survey of practices among gynaecologists in the British Isles. *Br J Obstet Gynaecol* **95**, 1178-89

Lockhart, J.L. *et al.* (1993) Anti-incontinence surgery in females with detrusor instability. *Proceedings of the Thirteenth Annual Meeting of the International Continence Society*, pp. 280-1. Aachen, Germany

Sand, P.K. *et al.* (1987) The low pressure urethra as a factor in failed retropubic urethropexy. *Obstet Gynecol* **160**, 452-8

Wilson, P.D. *et al.* (1987) An objective assessment of physiotherapy for female genuine stress incontinence. *Br J Obstet Gynaecol* **94**, 575-82

25 **With regard to microinvasive carcinoma of the cervix, which of the following statements are correct?**

A) It should not invade more than 5 mm below the surface of the epithelium.	FALSE
B) It will not spread horizontally more than 5 mm.	FALSE
C) It is best treated by hysterectomy.	FALSE
D) It cannot be diagnosed if it is incompletely excised.	TRUE
E) It cannot be diagnosed if lymph channels are involved.	FALSE

COMMENTS

Although a variety of definitions of microinvasive carcinoma of the cervix have been used in the past, FIGO recommend (Creasman 1987) that these be classified as: Ia1–minimal stromal invasion, and Ia2 – invasion depths of less than 5 mm from the base of the epithelium with a horizontal spread of no more than 7 mm. The diagnosis is usually made at cone biopsy; if excision is incomplete the dimensions cannot be measured. Cone biopsy is usually adequate treatment. Local excision is complete and lymph node metastasis is very uncommon. If lymph channel involvement is absent then nodal involvement is only seen in lesions nearer the 5 mm limit (approximately 3% nodal metastases). When lymph channels are involved the risk of node metastasis is related to the depth of invasion, less than 3% when the depth of invasion is 3 mm, but up to 10% when between 3–5 mm. In these latter cases further treatment may be prudent, but this would involve pelvic node dissection or radiotherapy; hysterectomy would confer no advantage (Duncan 1991).

REFERENCES

Creasman, W.T. (1987) Changes in FIGO staging. *Obstet Gynecol* **70**, 138

Duncan, I.D. (1991) The management of microinvasive carcinoma of the cervix. *Curr Obstet Gynaecol* **1**: 3, 143-6

26 Partial hydatidiform mole is:

A) A variety of trophoblastic disease in which the histological appearance is intermediate between that of classical hydatidiform mole and hydropic degeneration seen in other spontaneous abortions.   FALSE

B) A condition in which part of the placenta has undergone molar degeneration and the remainder is macroscopically and histologically normal.   FALSE

C) A condition in which a fetus may be found along with a placenta showing molar change.   TRUE

D) A condition which can be distinguished from complete mole cytogenically.   TRUE

E) Complicated by the development of persistent or invasive trophoblastic disease much less than following complete mole.   TRUE

COMMENTS

The histological changes in an aborted placenta may be difficult to interpret and some pathologists have described a transition from simple hydropic change to hydatidiform mole with only an arbitrary line of demarcation. At both ends of the spectrum macroscopic vesicles may be seen. The diagnostic criterion for complete mole should be the presence of trophoblastic hyperplasia.

Although the changes described above may be localised, when there are two distinct parts to a placenta – one normal with a fetus, and the other showing molar degeneration, the most likely explanation is a twin conception. The term 'partial hydatidiform mole' should be confined to an abnormal conceptus in which an embryo or fetus is recognisable with a placenta showing molar degeneration with focal trophoblastic hyperplasia. In some cases the only evidence of the embryo is that fetal nucleate red blood cells can be seen in the villous vessels.

It is now recognised that these pregnancies are triploid, commonly 69 XXY. This condition may be more common than complete mole but is not recognised as often because of the inadequate examination of aborted material. True choriocarcinoma is a rare sequel of partial mole but persistent invasive disease does occur and about 1% require chemotherapy (compared with some 6-10% after complete mole). Partial moles require registration and follow-up.

APPROPRIATE READING

Bagshawe, K.D., Lawler, S.D., Paradinas, P.J. *et al.* (1990) Gestational trophoblastic tumours following initial diagnosis of partial hydatidiform mole. *Lancet* **335**, 1074-6

Fox, H. (Ed.) (1978) *Pathology of the Placenta*, p. 265; Chapter 14. London: W.B. Saunders

World Health Organisation (1983) *Gestational Trophoblastic Tumours*. WHO Technical Report Series 692. London: HMSO

27 Dysgerminoma of ovary:

A) Is common below the age of 30.	TRUE
B) Produces alphafetoprotein (AFP).	FALSE
C) Is associated with gonadal dysgenesis.	TRUE
D) Is radio-sensitive.	TRUE
E) Recurs late, over ten years.	FALSE

COMMENTS

Dysgerminoma commonly arises in patients aged between ten and 30 years old (Scully 1979). Endodermal sinus tumour and embryonal carcinoma produce AFP but not dysgerminoma.

Dysgerminoma has a particular tendency to develop in patients with developmental abnormalities of the gonads (Scully 1979). Dysgerminoma is radio-sensitive (Thomas *et al.* 1987).

About 75% of recurrences occur within the first year after initial treatment (Slayton 1984). Granulosa cell tumours tend to occur late.

REFERENCES

Scully, R.E. (1979) Tumors of the ovary and maldeveloped gonads. *Atlas of Tumour Pathology* **Fascicle 16**. Washington, DC: Armed Forces Institute of Pathology

Slayton, R.E. (1984) Management of germ cell and stromal tumors of the ovary. *Semin Oncol* **11**, 299-313

Thomas, G.M., Dembo, A.J., Hacker, N.F. *et al.* (1987) Current therapy for dysgerminoma of the ovary. *Obstet Gynecol* **70** 268-75

28 In hormone replacement therapy (HRT):

A) Long-term usage has been conclusively demonstrated not to be associated with an increased risk of breast carcinoma. **FALSE**

B) Mortality is increased overall in HRT users over non-users. **FALSE**

C) Bisphosphonates (e.g. etidronate, clodronate) are indicated for the treatment and/or prevention of postmenopausal osteoporosis in patients in whom hormonal replacement therapy is contraindicated. **TRUE**

D) Placebo therapy is as effective as HRT in the treatment of hot flushes. **FALSE**

E) Flushes are cured by the abolition of elevated gonadotrophin levels due to negative feedback of exogenous oestradiol on pituitary LH secretion. **FALSE**

COMMENTS

There is a continuing lack of consensus on the effect of HRT on breast cancer risk. Some studies (Hoover *et al.* 1981; Brinton *et al.* 1986; Ewertz 1988) have reported a moderately increasing relative risk of 1.3–1.9 after 15-20 years' use. Others did not (Kaufman *et al.* 1984; Wingo *et al.* 1987). Data from 20-year follow-up in the American Nurses Health Study (Colditz *et al.* 1990) show no increased risk with long-term previous usage, although risk was increased with current usage, especially in older age groups.

Data from Hunt *et al.* (1990), updating a prospective cohort study of long-term HRT users, showed an increase in breast cancer mortality with increasing intervals since first exposure to HRT; in contrast to a decreased overall mortality from cardiovascular disease, though the relative risk was still unity compared to a previously reduced risk. Overall mortality is significantly lower than expected on the basis of national rates from other causes including endometrial cancer and cardiovascular disease.

Several therapies are available for osteoporosis which do not have a hormonal component, and act either by inhibiting osteoclast mediated bone resorption (calcium, calcitonin, bisphosphonates, and Vitamin D – secondarily by increasing calcium absorption), or stimulating osteoblast mediated bone formation (sodium fluoride, parathyroid hormone, amino-acid fragments, growth factors, calcitrol and exercise, as well as the non-oestrogenic anabolic steroids and testosterone). Bisphosphonates 'chemisorb' to bone crystal, so preventing osteoclast access for bone resorption. The activity and number of osteoclasts is also decreased. The net effect is to stabilise bone mass. Use should be intermittent rather than continuous to avoid potential mineralisation defects in bone resulting from reduced bone remodelling. Side effects are few; mild diarrhoea has been noted (Chesnut 1991).

Although there is undoubtedly a placebo effect in the treatment of hot flushes, two well-known, placebo-controlled, double-blind studies demonstrate a clear benefit from oestrogen therapy in the treatment of flushes (Coupe *et al.* 1975; Campbell and Whitehead 1977).

The endocrine events responsible for flushing remain poorly understood, but it has been shown that women unable to secrete LH flush (Meldrum *et al.* 1981) and that LHRH superagonists do not abolish flushing (Lightman *et al.* 1982).

REFERENCES

Brinton, L., Hoover, R.N. and Fraumeni, J.F. (1986) Menopausal oestrogens and breast cancer risk: an expanded case control study. *Br J Cancer* **54**, 825-32

Campbell, S. and Whitehead, M. (1977) Oestrogen therapy and the menopausal syndrome. *Clin Obstet Gynaecol* **4**, 31-47

Chesnut, C.H. (1991) Alternatives to sex steroids in osteoporosis. *Clin Obstet Gynaecol* **5**: 4, 857-65

Colditz, G.A., Stampfer, M.J., Willett, W.C. *et al.* (1990) Prospective study of oestrogen replacement therapy and risk of breast cancer in postmenopausal women. *JAMA* **264**, 2648-53

Coope, J., Thompson, J.M. and Poller, L. (1975) Effects of 'natural oestrogen' replacement therapy on menopausal symptoms and blood clotting. *BMJ* **4**, 139-43

Ewertz, M. (1988) Influence of non-contraceptive exogenous and endogenous sex hormones on breast cancer risk in Denmark. *Int J Cancer* **41**, 832-8

Hoover, R., Glass, A., Finkle, W.D. *et al.* (1981) Conjugated oestrogens and breast cancer risk. *J Nat Cancer Inst* **67**, 815-20

Hunt, K., Vessey, M. and McPherson, K. (1990) Mortality in a cohort of long-term users of hormone replacement therapy: an updated analysis. *Br J Obstet Gynaecol* **97**, 1080-5

Kaufman, D.W., Miller, D.R., Rosenberg, L. *et al.* (1984) Non-contraceptive estrogen use and the risk of breast cancer. *JAMA* **252**, 1, 63-7

Lightman, S.L., Jacobs, H.S. and Maguire, A.K. (1982) Down-regulation of gonadotrophin secretion in postmenopausal women by a superactive LHRH analogue: lack of effect on menopausal flushing. *Br J Obstet Gynaecol* **89**, 977-80

Meldrum, D.R., Erlik, Y., Lu, J.K. *et al.* (1981) Objectively recorded hot flushes in patients with pituitary insufficiency. *J Clin Endocrinol Metab* **49**, 152-4

Wingo, P.A., Layde, P.M. and Lee, N.C. (1987) The risk of breast cancer in postmenopausal women who have used oestrogen replacement therapy. *JAMA* **257**, 209-15

29 In severe ovarian hyperstimulation syndrome (OHSS):

A) Pleural effusion may occur.   TRUE
B) Intravascular clotting can be a complication.   TRUE
C) Hypoproteinaemia may develop.   TRUE
D) Bilateral oophorectomy is indicated.   FALSE
E) Pregnancy is uncommon.   FALSE

COMMENTS

Ovarian hyperstimulation syndrome (OHSS) may occur in women undergoing ovarian stimulation using gonadotrophins despite careful monitoring of the follicular phase. Schenker and Weinstein (1978) report an up to 10% incidence of severe OHSS in women undergoing stimulation with human menopausal gonadrotrophin (HMG) while Golan et al. (1988) found an incidence of 8.4% in women who had long-acting GnRH agonist and HMG.

The exact aetiology and pathogenesis is unknown despite numerous investigations but the condition correlates well with large numbers of follicles or corpora lutea and high levels of 17-beta oestradiol and progesterone and it is invariably precipitated by HCG used for ovulation induction and that of embryonic origin. Women who present with ovarian hyperstimulation a few days after undergoing embryo replacement should be strongly suspected of being pregnant. Hack et al. (1970) reported a 6% incidence of severe OHSS in patients who had conceived after ovulation induction using HCG. Tyler (1968) observed some type of OHSS in 50% of patients during the cycle in which conception occurred resulting from ovulation induction.

Clinically, the syndrome manifests itself with abdominal distension and pain of varying intensity. Ovarian enlargement occurs and the ovaries are often palpable well above the symphysis pubis. Patients may be dyspnoeic due to abdominal distension (caused by transudation of protein and oestrogen-rich fluid into the peritoneal cavity) and/or pleural effusion. There is accompanying hypovolaemia, reduced urinary output, hypoproteinaemia and electrolyte imbalance and intravascular clotting may occur (Schenker and Weinstein 1978).

The management of severe ovarian hyperstimulation is essentially conservative and treatment is directed to correcting hypovolaemia and maintaining urinary output and appropriate electrolyte replacement. In cases where intravascular clotting occurs heparin treatment may be required. Paracentesis and tapping of pleural effusions may be necessary and only rarely is laparotomy necessary for torsion of an ovary or to control haemorrhage. The surgery should be conservative (Schenker and Weinstein 1978).

Severe ovarian hyperstimulation may be avoided in women who are down-regulated with GnRH analogues who have multiple follicular development and markedly elevated levels of 17-beta oestradiol by avoiding the administration of HCG, withdrawing stimulation with gonadotrophins and maintaining pituitary desensitisation until the onset of menstruation (Shaw and Amso 1989).

REFERENCES

Golan, A., Ron-El, R., Herman, A. et al. (1988) Ovarian hyperstimulation syndrome following D-Trp-6 luteinising hormone-releasing microcapsules and menotropin for in vitro fertilisation. Fertil Steril 50: 6, 912-16

Hack, M., Brish, M., Serr, D.M. et al. (1970) Outcome of pregnancies after induced ovulation. J Am Med Assoc 211, 791-7

Schenker, J.G. and Weinstein, D. (1978) Ovarian hyperstimulation syndrome: a current survey. Fertil Steril 30, 3, 255-68

Shaw, R.W. and Amso, N. (1989) 'New concepts in GnRH associated superovulation for polycystic ovary syndrome in assisted reproduction programs' in Chronic Hyperandrogenic Anovulation. Carnforth: Parthenon Publishing

Tyler, E.T. (1968) Treatment of anovulation with menotropins. J Am Med Assoc 205, 86-92

30 **The action of progestogens on the endometrial cell include:**

A) Reduction of oestrone levels.   FALSE
B) Reduction of oestradiol levels.   TRUE
C) Reduction of oestradiol-17 beta dehydrogenase activity.   FALSE
D) Reduction of oestrogen receptor.   TRUE
E) Reduction of progesterone receptor.   TRUE

COMMENTS

Within the endometrium progestogens oppose the proliferative effects of oestrogen. The levels of oestradiol, which is the most potent oestrogen, are significantly reduced (King *et al.* 1980) but oestrone levels remain unchanged (Whitehead *et al.* 1981). Oestradiol is converted to oestrone by oestradiol-17 beta dehydrogenase, the activity of which is increased by progestogen treatment (King *et al.* 1981). Oestrone is presumably then lost from within the cell.

Another way in which progestogens may oppose the stimulatory activity of oestrogens on the endometrium is to reduce the amount of available oestrogen receptor and therefore prevent the active hormone from reaching the endometrial cell nucleus (Pollow *et al.* 1980). Progestogens paradoxically also reduce the formation of their own receptor proteins (Levy *et al.* 1980).

REFERENCES

King, R.J., Dyer, G., Collins, W.P. *et al.* (1980) Intracellular estradiol, estrone and estrogen receptor levels in endometria from postmenopausal women receiving estrogens and progestins. *J Steroid Biochem* **13**, 4, 377-82

King, R.J., Townsend, P.T. and Whitehead, M.I. (1981) The role of estradiol dehydrogenase in mediating progestin effects on endometrium from postmenopausal women receiving estrogens and progestins. *J Steroid Biochem* **14**, 3, 235-8

Levy, C., Robel, P., Gautray, J.P. *et al.* (1980) Estradiol and progesterone receptors in human endometrium: normal and abnormal menstrual cycles and early pregnancy. *Am J Obstet Gynecol* **136**, 646-51

Pollow, K., Schmidt-Gollwitzer, M. and Pollow, B. (1980) 'Progesterone- and estradiol-binding proteins from normal human endometrium and endometrial carcinoma: a comparative study' in J.L. Wittliff and O. Dapunt (Eds) *Steroid Receptors and Hormone Dependent Neoplasia*, pp. 69-94. New York: Masson Publishing

Whitehead, M.I., Lane, G., Dyer, G. *et al.* (1981) Oestradiol: the predominant intranuclear oestrogen in the endometrium of oestrogen treated postmenopausal women. *Br J Obstet Gynaecol* **88**, 914-18

31 Which of the following statements regarding female sexual disorders are correct?

A) Fifty per cent of patients present with orgasmic dysfunction. FALSE
B) Non-organic type I dyspareunia responds to education and systematic desensitisation. TRUE
C) Combined oral contraceptive pill is associated with impaired sexual dysfunction. FALSE
D) A woman who has recently lost interest in sex could be defined as having secondary situational impaired sexual desire. FALSE
E) Secretory pituitary prolactinoma is associated with impaired sexual dysfunction. TRUE

COMMENTS

Impaired sexual desire is the most common presentation in women to sexual dysfunction clinics. Orgasmic dysfunction accounts for 20% of presenting women (Hawton 1984).

Dyspareunia may be caused by organic or non-organic factors. Non-organic type I dyspareunia is diagnosed when the presentation involves guilt, misinformation or previous traumatic experiences, and type II where marital problems and poor communication lead to dyspareunia being used as an excuse to avoid sex (Mira 1988).

Combined oral contraceptive pill has been linked to impaired sexual desire but studies are inconclusive (Cullberg 1973). Pituitary adenoma with hyperprolactinaemia is associated with impaired sexual arousal.

Impaired sexual desire can be primary or secondary, total or situational. For example, a woman who has never had interest in sex would be said to have primary total impaired sexual desire, whereas a woman who has lost her interest in sex with her husband whilst having no problems with her lover could be defined as having secondary situational impaired sexual desire.

REFERENCES

Cullberg, J. (1973) Mood changes and menstrual symptoms with different gestagen/estrogen combinations. A double-blind comparison with a placebo. *Acta Psychiatr Scand* (Suppl) **236**, 1-86

Hawton, K. (1984) *Sex Therapy: A Practical Guide*. Oxford: Oxford University Press

Mira, J.J. (1988) A therapeutic package for dyspareunia: a three case example. *Sex Marital Ther* **3**: 1, 77-82

32 Non-contraceptive benefits of combined oral contraceptives include:

A) Prevention of pregnancy.	FALSE
B) Treatment of menstrual dysfunction.	TRUE
C) Reduction in the risk of pelvic inflammatory disease (PID).	TRUE
D) Protection against ovarian cancer.	TRUE
E) Protection against cervical but not against endometrial cancer.	FALSE

COMMENTS

The primary action of combined oral contraceptives (COCs) is to suppress the mid-cycle gonadotrophin surge and this results in inhibition of ovulation. Oral contraceptives also suppress episodic gonadotrophin release such that ovarian steroidogenesis is reduced. Prevention of pregnancy is a contraceptive benefit of COCs. In addition to prevention of pregnancy, COCs have both adverse and many non-contraceptive benefits (Connell 1987). When menorrhagia exists, there is usually irregular shedding of the endometrium, either in the presence or absence of ovulation.

If the bleeding is prolonged, anaemia may result acutely or gradually. The use of COCs stabilises the endometrium, inducing a constant dysynchrony between glands and stroma. Mishell (1982) showed that COCs halved the prevalence of menorrhagia, inter-menstrual bleeding and irregular periods. The same study also demonstrated a 50% reduction in the frequency of iron deficiency anaemia and a 40% reduction in primary dysmenorrhoea. The incidence of PID is significantly reduced in women receiving COCs (Higgins et al. 1985). Reduction in menstrual flow in COC users is regarded as a factor in minimising exposure of the reproductive tract to infectious organisms. Oral contraceptives also make cervical mucus thicker and less penetrable to bacteria. Because COCs suppress follicular development and ovulation, there is a reduction in the occurrence of functional ovarian cysts (Vessey et al. 1987) and at least 12 studies have concluded that COCs protect women from ovarian cancer (Cancer and Steroid Hormone Study 1987a; Khoo 1986). A decrease in the risk of endometrial cancer has been noted by at least ten studies (Cancer and Steroid Hormone Study 1987b). On the other hand, it would appear that COC users may actually have an increased risk of developing cervical cancer (Beral et al. 1988). In the latter case, other factors such as multiple partners, high risk male partner and sexually transmitted infections are contributory.

Combined oral contraceptives have important non-contraceptive benefits, especially protection against ovarian and endometrial cancer. Unfortunately the over-publicity of the adverse effects of COCs by the media has affected the uptake of COCs by teenagers who are most at risk of unplanned pregnancy and for whom other contraceptive methods are unsuitable.

REFERENCES

Beral, V., Jamaford, P. and Kay, C. (1988) Oral contraceptives and malignancies of the genital tract. *Lancet* **ii**, 1331-4

Cancer and Steroid Hormone Study of the Centres for Disease Control and the National Institute of Child Health and Human Development (1987a) The reduction in risk of ovarian cancer associated with oral contraceptive use. *N Engl J Med* **316**, 650-5

Cancer and Steroid Hormone Study of the Centres for Disease Control and the National Institute of Child Health and Human Development (1987b) Combination oral contraceptive use and the risk of endometrial cancer. *JAMA* **257**, 796-800

Connell, E.B. (1987) Oral contraceptives: the benefits and the cardiovascular risks. *Postgrad Med* **81**, 46-58

Higgins, J.E., Wilkens, L.R., Chi, I.C. *et al.* (1985) Hospitalizations among black women using contraceptives. *Am J Obstet Gynecol* **153**, 3, 280-7

Khoo, S.K. (1986) Cancer risk and the contraceptive pill. *Med J Aust* **144**, 185-90

Mishell, D.R. (1982) Non-contraceptive health benefits of steroidal contraceptives. *Am J Obstet Gynecol* **142**, 809-16

Vessey, M., Metcalfe, A., Wells, C. *et al.* (1987) Ovarian neoplasm, functional ovarian cysts, and oral contraceptives. *BMJ* **294**, 1518-20

33 Endometrial cancer:

A) Is more common in women using oestrogens and progestogens for hormone replacement therapy.   FALSE
B) Is staged clinically prior to definitive treatment by examination under anaesthetic and fractional curettage.   FALSE
C) May exhibit secretory changes in response to progestogens.   TRUE
D) Survival improves if surgery is preceded by pelvic radiotherapy.   FALSE
E) May be treated successfully by Heyman's Capsules.   TRUE

COMMENTS

It is now well established that in women who use oestrogens in combination with progestogens, endometrial cancer is less common (Persson *et al.* 1986). The clinical (1971) FIGO staging of endometrial cancer was replaced in 1988, since when the disease has been surgically staged following definitive surgery as follows:

Stage	IA G123	Tumour limited to endometrium
	IB G123	Invasion to < half myometrium
	IC G123	Invasion to > half myometrium
Stage	IIA G123	Endocervical glandular involvement only
	IIB G123	Cervical stromal invasion
Stage	IIIA G123	Tumour invades serosa and/or adnexa and/or positive peritoneal cytology
	IIIB G123	Vaginal metastases
	IIIC G123	Metastases to pelvic and/or para-aortic lymph nodes
Stage	IVA G123	Tumour invasion of bladder and/or bowel mucosa
	IVB	Distant metastases including intra-abdominal metastases and/or inguinal lymph nodes

(G123 is the histological grading of the tumour.)

If progestogens are used prior to definitive surgery secretory changes may occur within the tumour (Ferenczy and Richart 1974).

There is no evidence to suggest that preoperative radiotherapy to the pelvis enhances survival in endometrial cancer. Women who are a poor operative risk may be treated successfully with Heyman's Capsules which are used to pack the endometrial cavity with a radioactive source.

REFERENCES

Ferenczy, A. and Richart, R.M. (1974) 'Endometrium associated with hyperestrogenic states' in *Female Reproductive System: Dynamics of Scan and Transmission Electron Microscopy*, pp. 154-61. New York: John Wiley

Persson, I.R., Adami, H-O, Ekund, G. *et al.* (1986) The risk of endometrial neoplasia and treatment with estrogens and estrogen-progestogen combinations. *Acta Obstet Gynecol Scand* **65**, 211-17

34 Which of the following statements with regard to the IUCD are correct?

A) Modern copper IUCDs are clinically effective and safe for at least five years.   TRUE

B) It reduces the number of sperm reaching the fallopian tube and their capacity to fertilise the egg.   TRUE

C) The risk of pelvic infection (PID) is low (<2 cases PID/ 1000 woman years of use) and does not increase with long-term use.   TRUE

D) Is contraindicated in women with Wilson's disease.   TRUE

E) Levonorgestrel releasing devices are associated with a highly significant reduction in blood loss in women with menorrhagia.   TRUE

COMMENTS

Long-term use of early copper IUCDs (Copper 7 and Copper T) was associated with fragmentation and even disappearance of the copper wire. Modern copper IUCDs have thicker wire, use silver-core copper wire or have solid copper collars or sleeves. The FPA and NAFPD issued a statement in 1990 advising that modern IUCDs could be left in place for five years (Newton and Tacchi 1990).

Whilst many doctors attribute the effectiveness of the IUD to the inhibition of implantation, there is significant evidence that it reduces both the number and viability of eggs and sperm (Sivin 1989). This is of relevance to international agencies providing family planning programmes, because there is a reluctance on the part of some governments to support the methods which might be seen as abortifications. The World Health Organisation recently published the results of a large multi-centre study involving almost 23 000 women using IUDs (Farley *et al.* 1992). The overall rate of PID was 1.6/1000 woman years of use but was increased more than six times during the first 20 days after insertion. Rates were lower in women who had recent insertions, suggesting that there may be a trend towards improving sterile techniques. The practical application of these findings is to encourage very careful aseptic techniques at the time of insertion.

The levonorgestrel (LNG) releasing IUCD (releasing 20 µg LNG/day) causes endometrial atrophy without altering ovarian function. Many women develop amenorrhoea and one study (Andersson and Rybo 1990) of women presenting with menorrhagia suggests that the IUCD may be a cheap and effective medical treatment for this common complaint.

REFERENCES

Andersson, K. and Rybo, G. (1990) Levonorgestrel releasing intrauterine device in the treatment of menorrhagia. *Br J Obstet Gynaecol* **97**, 690-4

Farley, T.M.M.M., Rosenberg, M.J., Rowe, P.J. *et al.* (1992) Intrauterine devices and pelvic inflammatory disease. An international perspective. *Lancet* **339**, 785-91

Newton, J. and Tacchi, D. (1990) Long-term use of copper intrauterine devices. *Lancet* **335**, 1322-3

Sivin, I. (1989) IUDs are contraceptives, not abortifacients: A comment on research and belief. *Stud Fam Plann* **20**, 355-9

35 Which of the following statements concerning endometriosis are correct?

A) In mild to moderate disease and in terms of reproductive outcome, hormonal manipulation has no benefit over expectant management. TRUE

B) Oestrogen and progestin receptor concentrations are similar in endometriotic lesions and in ectopic endometrium. FALSE

C) These receptor concentrations increase with the severity of the endometriotic lesions. FALSE

D) Presurgical hormonal manipulation will usually decrease the size of endometriotic cysts and increase the ease of surgery. FALSE

E) Hormone replacement therapy can be started immediately after surgery for endometriosis. TRUE

COMMENTS

There are data to suggest that medroxyprogesterone acetate (30 mg daily) may be just as good as danazol in terms of affecting reproductive outcome but that neither has an advantage over expectant management in mild or moderate disease.

In the study by Janne *et al.* (1981) cytosol oestrogen and progestin levels were compared in endometriotic lesions and in endometrial tissue. Half of the endometriosis specimens contained progestin receptors only and in concentrations significantly lower than in equivalent endometrial specimens. In addition, whilst oestrogen and progestin receptors were measurable in the majority of endometrial samples, both were present in only 40% of endometriosis specimens.

There are no data to show that the severity of endometriotic lesions exerts any effect on receptor concentrations. Medical treatment seems to have little effect on the size of endometriotic deposits and since the majority of surgical problems encountered in patients with endometriosis relate to tissue destruction, scarring and adhesions rather than active endometriosis, it would be fanciful to believe that hormonal manipulation would exert any significant influence on eventual surgery (Hull *et al.* 1986). In one study, Henderson and Studd (1991) concluded that HRT could be started immediately after surgery for endometriosis and would not lead to reactivation of the disease. However, in this study HRT consisted of oestrogen implants combined with testosterone and the latter may have had an effect on the disease. The authors, however, claimed that the dose of testosterone was too low to exert any significant androgenic effect. Nevertheless, the anxieties about oestrogen HRT alone in women with endometriosis must remain.

REFERENCES

Henderson, A.F. and Studd, J. (1991) 'The role of definitive surgery and hormone replacement therapy in the treatment of endometriosis' in E.J. Thomas and J. Rock (Eds) *Modern Approaches to Endometriosis*, pp. 275-90. London: Kluwer Academic

Hull, M.E., Moghissi, K.S., Magyar, D.F. *et al.* (1986) Comparison of different treatment modalities of endometriosis in infertile women. *Fertil Steril* **47**, 40-4

Janne, O., Kauppila, A., Kokko, E. *et al.* (1981) Estrogen and progestin receptors in endometriotic lesions: comparison with endometrial tissue. *Am J Obstet Gynecol* **141**, 562-6

FURTHER READING

Thomas, E.J. (1992) Combining medical and surgical treatments for endometriosis: the best of both worlds? *Br J Obstet Gynaecol* **99** (suppl. 7), 5-8

36 **Surgical management is the treatment of choice for genuine stress incontinence. Which of the following statements are correct?**

A) The success for vaginal repair operations after two years is 85%.   FALSE
B) The Burch colposuspension operation approximates the paravaginal tissue to the ipsilateral iliopectineal ligament.   TRUE
C) Sling procedures are associated with a high incidence of complications.   TRUE
D) Stamey bladder neck suspension is the operation of choice in elderly patients with incontinence.   TRUE
E) Previous bladder neck surgery is a poor prognostic factor in subsequent management.   TRUE

COMMENTS

Early reviews of vaginal surgery in the control of stress incontinence demonstrated a highly satisfactory cure rate of 80-90% (Green 1975; Warrell 1986). However, the majority of authors have shown a much less encouraging result and improvement in control after two years has been as low as 30%. Randomised comparative studies demonstrate that elevation of the bladder neck by a suprapubic approach is preferable to vaginal surgery (Stanton and Cardozo 1979; Park and Millar 1988).

The Burch colposuspension operation achieves its effect by elevating the bladder neck, increasing the intra-abdominal length of the urethra, increasing the posterior vesico-vaginal angle and reducing the internal diameter of the urethra. This is achieved by suturing the paravaginal tissues to the iliopectineal ligament on the same side (Ashkers et al. 1984).

The indication for suburethral sling procedures is failure of previous surgical procedures and as a result damage to the bladder is more common. The use of foreign materials in the slings (teflon gauze, silastic) lead to rejection, sinus and abcess formation.

The Stamey procedure (Stamey 1973) does not involve dissection and so complications are fewer and postoperative recovery more rapid. It is suited to elderly and infirm patients but may also be indicated in some patients with previous failure because of the lack of dissection.

Scarring from previous surgery not only renders future surgery more difficult but it adversely influences the success of future attempts to correct the complaint.

Endoscopic techniques with injection of collagen (Eckford and Abrams 1991) may offer an improvement in those situations. Teflon (Politano et al. 1974) has, however, lost popularity because of a decline in success with the passage of time and fear of embolisation.

REFERENCES

Ashkers, M.H., Abrams, P.H. and Lawrence, W.T. (1984) Stamey endoscopic bladder neck suspension for stress urinary incontinence. *Br J Urol* **56**, 629-34

Eckford, S.D. and Abrams, P.H. (1991) Para-urethral collagen implantation for female stress incontinence. *Br J Urol* **68**, 586-9

Green, T.H. (1975) Urinary stress incontinence; differential diagnosis, pathophysiology and management. *Am J Obstet Gynecol* **122**, 368-400

Keane, D.P. and Eckford, S.D. (1992) Surgical treatment of urinary stress incontinence. *Br J Hosp Med* **48**, 308-13

Park, G.S. and Millar, E.J. (1988) Surgical treatment of stress urinary incontinence; comparison of the Kelly plication, Marshall-Marchetti-Kranz and Pereyra procedures. *Obstet Gynecol* **71**, 575-9

Politano, V.A., Small, M.P., Harper, J.M. et al. (1974) Periurethral Teflon injection for urinary incontinence. *J Urol* **111**, 180-3

Stamey, T.A. (1973) Endoscopic suspension of the vesical neck for urinary incontinence. *Surg Gynaecol Obstet* **136**, 547-54

Stanton, S.L. and Cardozo, L.D. (1979) A comparison of vaginal and suprapubic surgery in the correction of incontinence due to urethral sphincter incompetence. *Br J Urol* **51** 497-9

Warrell, D. (1986) 'Anterior repair' in S.L. Stanton and E.A. Tenagho (Eds) *Surgery for Female Incontinence*, pp. 77-86. Berlin: Springer-Verlag

37 Tuboperitoneal disorders may occur as a result of salpingitis, endometriosis or previous abdomino-pelvic surgery. The success of tuboplasty is dependent upon the degree of original inflammatory damage, the site of tubal closure, the causative pathogen and the postoperative length of viable tube. Which of the following statements are correct?

A) Proximal lesions of the fallopian tube occur less often than lesions of the distal end.   FALSE
B) Endometriosis is a cause of non-obliterative disease.   TRUE
C) Hydrosalpinx formation is frequently associated with extensive lesions of the mucosa.   TRUE
D) Motile cilia are essential for conception.   FALSE
E) Surgical correction of distal occlusion can result in a pregnancy rate of approximately 30% after two years.   TRUE

COMMENTS

Tubal peritoneal disorders are variously reported in the literature as accounting for some 12-35% of causes of infertility in women. The major early event of reproduction, oocyte transfer, the final phases of sperm transport and capacitation, fertilisation and embryo transport all take place in the tubal lumen and are dependent upon different aspects of tubal function which in turn relate to normal tubal architecture.

Peri-tubal and peri-ovarian adhesions, tubal occlusion and endosalpingeal destruction give rise to infertility and also appear to be relevant to the outcome of tubal surgery, with the exception of those with immotile but otherwise normal cilia.

Recent publications have reawakened the debate of IVF as a surgery for this group of women with tuboperitoneal disease. The results, however, are seen to vary between specialist and non-specialist units. Undoubtedly the results of reconstructive surgery of the distal tube are less promising than correction of proximal occlusion, the latter having reported live birth rates of 40-60%.

Most instances of distal tubal occlusion are associated with an ascending genital tract infection and are to a lesser degree the result of pelvic peritonitis or iatrogenic surgical influences. They are more likely to have severe endosalpingeal damage and consequently a poor prognosis.

The outcome of tubal surgery is related to many variables reflecting the extent and severity of pre-existing disease. Various classification systems have been reported in the literature, e.g. Hulka 1982; Boer-Meisel et al. 1986. The latter highlighted the importance of five factors for the prediction of subsequent conception rates in patients treated for hydrosalpinges combining the four most promising factors: the extent and nature of adhesions, the macroscopic condition of the endosalpinx and the thickness of the tubal wall.

Pregnancy is mainly associated with a normal endosalpinx; where there are many fixed adhesions and a thick tubal wall pregnancy failure is common.

The results of tubal microsurgery are difficult to express. Many would claim endoscopic salpingolysis and salpingostomy has equal success. Brosens (1987) reported using a rigid 3 mm telescope passed down the channel of the operating laparoscope, enabling him to assess the mucosa of the infundibulum and ampullary segments, the fallopian tube being distended by a saline solution. Video-salpingoscopy (tuboscopy) enables direct vision of the mucosal folds, allowing observation of mucosal lesions, e.g. flattened major folds, agglutination or complete loss. It does not, however, allow visualisation of the intramural and isthmic portions of the fallopian tube. The recent development of a very fine (0.3 mm) flexible falloposcope has enabled transuterine visualisation of this section of the fallopian tube which was hitherto out of reach (Corfman 1990).

Tubal endoscopy may help to refine the indications for tubal microsurgery or *in vitro* fertilisation and may also aid the selection of patients for intratubal transfer of gametes/embryos. It has now become possible to examine almost every aspect of the female reproductive tract *in vivo* using an endoscopic approach.

REFERENCES

Boer-Meisel, M.E., TeVelde, E.R., Habbema, J.D. *et al.* (1986) Predicting the pregnancy outcome in patients treated for hydrosalpinx: a prospective study. *Fertil Steril* **45**, 23-9

Brosens, I.A., Boeckx, W., Delattin, P.H. *et al.* (1987) Salpingoscopy: a new preoperative diagnostic tool in tubal infertility? *Br J Obstet Gynaecol* **94**, 722-8

Corfman, R.S. (1990) Falloposcopy: frontiers realised, a fantastic voyage revisited. *Fertil Steril* **54**: 4, 574-6

Hulka, J.K. (1982) Adnexal lesions: a prognostic staging and classification system based on a five-year survey of fertility surgery at Chapel Hill, North Carolina. *Am J Obstet Gynecol* **144**: 2, 141-7

FURTHER READING

Brosens, I.A. and Gordon, A.G. (1989) *Tubal Infertility*. London: Gower Medical Publishing

Gordon, A.G. and Lewis, B.V. (Eds) (1988) *Gynaecological Endoscopy*. London: Chapman and Hall Medical

Reis, H. (1991) Management of tubal infertility in the 1990s. *Br J Obstet Gynaecol* **98**, 619-23

38   Which of the following statements regarding hormone replacement therapy are correct?

A) Combined HRT is cardio-protective.   FALSE

B) Meta analysis of the published studies estimates that the reduction in the risk of coronary heart disease, attributable to oestrogen therapy, is 45%.   TRUE

C) There is compelling evidence to suggest that there are factors other than HRT which are important for achieving a significant reduction in the incidence of myocardial infarction.   TRUE

D) Bone densitometry provides an effective screening test for the risk of hip and vertebral fractures.   FALSE

E) Ten years of hormone replacement therapy appears to increase slightly the risk of breast cancer.   TRUE

COMMENTS

The majority of epidemiological studies (Meade and Berra 1992) reporting cardiovascular protection have been performed with natural oestrogens alone rather than with oestrogen plus progestogen (opposed therapy). Stampfer and Colditz (1991) estimated an overall reduction in the risk of coronary disease of 45%.

Within six months of the cessation of menstrual bleeding, there are increases of serum concentration of total cholesterol (by about 6%), low-density lipoprotein cholesterol (by about 11%) and triglycerides (by about 9%), together with a gradual fall in the high-density lipoprotein cholesterol concentration. With the exception of triglycerides, this atherogenic profile is reversed by treatment with oestrogen. The addition of progestogens blocks the oestrogen-induced increase of the cardio-protective, high-density lipoproteins.

Manson *et al.* (1992) have proposed that cessation of smoking, reduction in serum cholesterol, treatment of hypertension, regular exercise and the maintenance of ideal body weight will lead to a significant reduction in the risk of myocardial infarction.

Osteoporosis is characterised by low bone density with micro-architectural deterioration and consequent increased risk of fracture. Multiple factors contribute to bone loss postmenopausally. There are no sensitive parameters to identify women with low bone mass and those who are prone to rapid bone loss after the menopause (Johnston *et al.* 1991).

There is much evidence to suggest that oestrogens are involved in the aetiology of breast cancer. Evidence from the published meta analysis shows that the relative risk of developing breast cancer is about 1.1 after ten years and is unlikely to exceed 1.3 (Jacobs and Loeffler 1992).

REFERENCES

Jacobs, H.S. and Loeffler, F.E. (1992) Postmenopausal hormone replacement therapy. *BMJ* **305**, 1403-8

Johnston, C.C., Slemenda, C.W. and Milton, L.J. III (1991) Clinical use of bone densitometry. *N Engl J Med* **324**, 1105-9

Manson, J.E., Tosteson, H., Ridkir, P.M. *et al.* (1992) The primary prevention of myocardial infarction. *N Engl J Med* **326**, 21, 1406-16

Meade, T.W. and Berra, A. (1992) Hormone replacement treatment and cardiovascular disease. *Br Med Bull* **48**, 276-308

Stampfer, M.J. and Colditz, G.A. (1991) Oestrogen replacement therapy and coronary heart disease: a quantitative assessment of the epidemiological. *Prev Med* **20**, 47-63

39 In abnormal uterine bleeding in adolescents:

A) Ovulatory dysfunction is a rare cause.	FALSE
B) In girls with severe menorrhagia coagulation disorder should be excluded.	TRUE
C) The commonest haematological disorder is von Willebrand's disease.	FALSE
D) Pregnancy complications should be excluded.	TRUE
E) Evaluation of the patient must include a pelvic examination.	FALSE

COMMENTS

Known causes of abnormal uterine bleeding include:

(a) Anatomic lesions (polyps, fibroids, haemangiomas, vaginal adenosis).

(b) Coagulation disorders (von Willebrand's disease, idiopathic thrombocytopaenic purpura, platelet defect, thalassaemia major).

(c) Pregnancy complications (threatened abortion, ectopic pregnancy, hydatidiform mole, retained products of conception).

(d) Infections (vaginitis/cervicitis).

(e) Systemic disease (adrenal disorders, diabetes mellitus, hepatic dysfunction, thyroid dysfunction).

(f) Exogenous hormones.

Despite the above list of possible pathological causes of abnormal uterine bleeding in adolescents, over 95% of cases are caused by anovulatory dysfunctional uterine bleeding due to slow maturation of the hypothalamic-pituitary-ovarian axis. The basic abnormality is failure of the positive feedback mechanisms necessary to initiate the LH surge and ovulation despite increased follicular oestrogen levels (Hertweck 1992; Edmonds 1989; Kustin and Rebar 1987). Prolonged oestrogen stimulation of the endometrium results in hyperplasia. Claesseus and Cowell (1981) showed in a nine-year review that 19% of girls presenting with acute menorrhagia/anaemia had a primary coagulation disorder. Cases with excessive bleeding/anaemia must therefore be evaluated for blood dyscrasias. Thrombocytopaenic purpura is the commonest haematological disorder in adolescents (Gidwani 1984). Since the young adolescent may not always volunteer history of sexual activity, pregnancy complications as a cause of abnormal bleeding must never be forgotten.

Pelvic examination in an adolescent can be both embarrassing and very distressing. With the availability of scans, vaginal or pelvic examination is rarely necessary in modern days. A pelvic scan will not only be diagnostic, but will be very reassuring to the patient and her parents. Since the adolescent has to undergo a lot of emotional, psychological and physical change, sympathetic and adequate management of abnormal uterine bleeding will help eliminate an extra source of distress.

REFERENCES

Claesseus, E.A. and Cowell, C.A. (1981) Acute adolescent menorrhagia. *Am J Obstet Gynecol* **139**, 277-82

Edmonds, D.K. (1989) *Menstrual Changes in Adolescence (Baillière's Clin Obstet Gynaecol)* **3**: 2, 329-39. London: Baillière Tindall

Gidwani, G.P. (1984) Vaginal bleeding in adolescents. *J Reprod Med* **29**: 6, 417-20

Hertweck, S.P. (1992) Dysfunctional uterine bleeding. *Obstet Gynecol Clin North Am* **19**: 1, 129-49

Kustin, J. and Rebar, R.W. (1987) Menstrual disorders in the adolescent age group. *Primary Care* **14**: 1, 139-66

40 Regarding danazol, which of the following statements are correct?

A) It has a therapeutic place in treating conditions which respond to an increase in gonadal steroid activity.   FALSE

B) Its effects are all achieved through actions on the hypothalamic-pituitary-gonadal axis.   FALSE

C) It increases the hepatic sex hormone binding globulin (SHBG) synthesis.   FALSE

D) A six-month course is usually sufficient for treating moderate/severe endometriosis.   TRUE

E) At doses of 100-400 mg/day over 2-4 months it relieves the pain and tenderness of severe cyclical mastalgia.   TRUE

COMMENTS

Danazol has a well-established therapeutic place in treating conditions which respond to a reduction in gonadal steroid activity. Its effects are achieved through actions on the hypothalamic-pituitary-gonadal axis, on the plasma disposition and bio-availability of testosterone and oestradiol, and on the target tissue response to endogenous gonadal steroids.

Danazol appears also to affect the immune responses. It is therefore a complex mode of action, the components of which probably vary in their significance according to the therapeutic application and dosage employed.

The clinical value of danazol was first recorded in the treatment of endometriosis in 1971 by Greenblatt *et al.* (1971).

Danazol suppresses the mid-cycle LH and FSH surges, reduces LH pulsatility and inhibits ovarian responsiveness and steroidogenesis. Hill *et al.* (1987) observed an immunosuppressive effect of danazol on macrophage dependent T-lymphocyte proliferation. Danazol decreases the level of SHBG by direct inhibition of its hepatic synthesis.

Six months is usually a sufficient course for treating moderate/severe endometriosis. A shorter period of time may prove inadequate, and a longer period of time, e.g. up to nine months, may be necessary in some cases. Dosage should be adjusted to individual patient response, amenorrhoea being a useful guide.

At doses of 100-400 mg/day over 2-4 months, danazol relieves the pain and tenderness of severe cyclical mastalgia. Improvement is likely to be sustained for several months after the treatment.

Acne, oily skin and increased facial hair are most likely to be experienced by brunettes with a disposition to such problems (Rakoff 1976).

Danazol has been used in the treatment of PMS; studies showed benefit over placebo with a high rate of drop out (Gilmore *et al.* 1985).

REFERENCES

Gilmore, D.H., Hawthorne, R.J. and Hart, D.M. (1985) Danol for premenstrual syndrome: a preliminary report of a placebo controlled double blind study. *J Int Med Res* **13**, 129-30

Greenblatt, R.B., Dmowski, W.P., Mahesh, V.B. *et al.* (1971) Clinical studies with an anti-gonadotrophin, danazol. *Fertil Steril* **22**, 102-12

Hill, J.A., Barbieri, R.L. and Anderson, D.J. (1987) Immunosuppressive effects of danazol *in vitro*. *Fertil Steril* **48**: 3, 414-18

Rakoff, A.E. (1976) Side effects of danazol therapy. *Int Congr Ser* **368**, 108-15

41 Around the time of the menopause:

A) A serum FSH concentration of 20 iu/l strongly suggests that a woman is past the menopause. FALSE

B) The pregnancy rate is 5 per 100 woman years at aged 50. TRUE

C) Women should be advised to continue contraception for one year after the menopause if it occurs after they are 50. TRUE

D) The upper age limit for use of the newer combined oral contraceptives in healthy non-smoking women is 40 years. FALSE

E) If a woman aged 50 years is on a progesterone-only pill and becomes amenorrhoeic, she need not continue contraception. FALSE

COMMENTS

The natural menopause is the final menstrual period (FMP). It is usually diagnosed retrospectively after 12 months' amenorrhoea (McKinlay *et al.* 1991). After the FMP serum oestrogen levels fall and pituitary gonadotrophin levels rise. A serum FSH concentration of more than 30 iu/l on two occasions indicates the woman is past the menopause.

If no contraception is used during the perimenopause the pregnancy rate is between 10 and 20 per 100 woman years at age 45 and up to 5 per 100 woman years at the age of 50 (*Drug and Therapeutics Bulletin* 1991). Pregnancy at this age is rarely welcome and even this low risk may be unacceptable. Therefore women are advised to continue contraception for one year after the FMP if it occurs after they are 50 and for two years if the FMP occurs earlier.

There is no upper age limit for use of the newer combined oral contraceptives in healthy non-smoking women (Fortney 1990). Women who use a progestogen-only pill (POP) generally have 'normal' menstrual cycles but some have amenorrhoea. The menopause should be suspected if amenorrhoea develops in a woman in her mid-40s whose cycles on the POP were previously regular. The POP does not suppress the rise in FSH at the menopause, so FSH levels can be used to confirm the menopause in a woman taking this form of contraception. Serum FSH levels should be measured if amenorrhoea occurs in a woman above the age of 40. If the FSH level is high (more than 30 iu/l) on two occasions separated by three months, the POP can be stopped but, once again, simple non-hormonal contraception such as the sponge should be used for 12 months (*Drug and Therapeutics Bulletin* 1992).

REFERENCES

Drug and Therapeutics Bulletin (1991) Oral contraception in the peri-menopause. *Drug Ther Bull* **29**, 1, 3-4

Drug and Therapeutics Bulletin (1992) Advice on contraception around the menopause. *Drug Ther Bull* **30**, 24, 95-6

Fortney, J.A. (1990) Oral contraceptives for older women. *IPFF Med Bull* **24**, 3-4

McKinlay, S.M., Bramilla, D.J., Avis, N.E. *et al.* (1991) Women's experience of the menopause. *Curr Obstet Gynaecol* **1**, 3-7

42 In women who have undergone hysterectomy, a subsequent diagnosis of vaginal intraepithelial neoplasia (VAIN) of the vault:

A) Suggests inadequate assessment at the time of primary surgery.	TRUE
B) Is rare in the face of normal histological examination of the uterus and cervix.	TRUE
C) Is more common in immunocompromised individuals.	TRUE
D) Should be treated by laser vaporisation.	FALSE
E) Often presents with dyspareunia.	FALSE

COMMENTS

Vaginal intraepithelial neoplasia (VAIN) is a rare and generally asymptomatic disorder which usually occurs as an extension of cervical disease. When the diagnosis is made in women who have previously undergone hysterectomy, histological examination of the original uterine specimen often reveals intraepithelial neoplasia at the surgical margins (Woodman *et al.* 1984). In the absence of a previous history of cervical atypia the incidence of subsequent VAIN is low and would not generally warrant continued cytological surveillance in hysterectomised women. Women with immune dysfunction have a higher incidence of multifocal genital tract disease (Sillman *et al.* 1984). Buried atypical epithelium at the vaginal vault may not be amenable to laser therapy whereas surgical excision of the vaginal vault will allow both the removal of disease and the exclusion of occult invasion (Ireland and Monaghan 1988).

REFERENCES

Ireland, D. and Monaghan, J.M. (1988) The management of the patient with abnormal vaginal cytology following hysterectomy. *Br J Obstet Gynaecol* **95**, 973-5

Sillman, F., Stanek, A., Sedlis, A. *et al.* (1984) The relationship between human papilloma virus and lower genital tract neoplasia in immunosuppressed women. *Am J Obstet Gynecol* **150**, 300-8

Woodman, C.B.J., Jordan, J.A. and Wade Evans, T. (1984) The management of VAIN after hysterectomy. *Br J Obstet Gynaecol* **91**, 707-11

43 In mild endometriosis and subfertility:

A) The relationship between mild endometriosis and infertility is well proven.   FALSE

B) There is evidence that mild endometriosis is associated with abnormal follicular development.   FALSE

C) Luteinised unruptured follicle syndrome (LUF) has been noted to be present in about 50% of women with mild endometriosis.   FALSE

D) Infertile women are 7–10 times more likely to have mild endometriosis than their fertile counterparts.   FALSE

E) Medical treatment of mild endometriosis enhances cumulative conception rates.   FALSE

COMMENTS

A plethora of uncontrolled studies suggests that mild endometriosis causes subfertility. The main reason for this suggestion appears to be, firstly, that endometriosis is relatively frequent among infertile women (21–48%) and, secondly, relatively infrequent among previously fertile women undergoing laparoscopic sterilisation (1–5%). However, a few recently published studies have reported an incidence of between 18% and 43% in previously fertile women (Mahmood and Templeton 1991a).

Data on follicular development and periovulatory endocrinology are inconsistent (Mahmood and Templeton 1990), but recently reported prospective studies report that most of the women with mild endometriosis exhibit normal folliculogenesis when compared to a controlled group of tubal infertility (Mahmood et al. 1991a, b; Thomas et al. 1986).

The data on LUF syndrome are not in agreement and the incidence varies between 4% and 34% (Mahmood and Templeton 1991b). Although uncontrolled studies have reported a significant enhancement in fertility, following medical and/or surgical treatment, controlled studies (Hull et al. 1987; Thomas and Cooke 1987; Bayer et al. 1988) did not report a pregnancy enhancing effect on medical treatment. Mahmood (1991) reported that prior medical treatment did not alter circulating hormonal levels, characteristics of an LH surge and follicular development.

REFERENCES

Bayer, S.R., Seibel, M.M., Saffan, D.S. et al. (1988) Efficacy of danazol treatment for minimal endometriosis in fertile women: a prospective randomized study. *J Reprod Med* **33**, 179-83

Hull, M.E., Moghissi, K.S., Magyar, D.F. and Hayes, M.F. (1987) Comparison of different treatment modalities of endometriosis in infertile women. *Fertil Steril* **47**, 40-4

Mahmood, T.A. (1991) The impact of previous danazol treatment on circulating hormone levels, follicular development and oocyte maturity in minimal-mild endometriosis. *Eur J Obstet Gynaecol Report Biol* **41**, 207-14

Mahmood, T.A. and Templeton, A. (1990) Pathophysiology of mild endometriosis: a review of literature. *Hum Reprod* **5**, 765-84

Mahmood, T.A. and Templeton, A. (1991a) Prevalence and genesis of endometriosis. *Hum Reprod* **6**, 544-9

Mahmood, T.A. and Templeton, A. (1991b) Folliculogenesis and ovulation in infertile women with mild endometriosis. *Hum Reprod* **6**, 227-31

Mahmood, T.A., Arumugam, K. and Templeton, A. (1991a) Oocytes and follicular fluid characteristics in women with mild endometriosis. *Br J Obstet Gynaecol* **98**, 573-7

Mahmood, T.A., Messinis, I.E. and Templeton, A. (1991b) Follicular development in spontaneous and stimulated cycles in women with minimal-mild endometriosis. *Br J Obstet Gynaecol* **98**, 783-8

Thomas, E.J. and Cooke, I.D. (1987) Successful treatment of asymptomatic endometriosis: does it benefit infertile women? *BMJ* **294**, 1117-19

Thomas, E.J., Lenton, E.A. and Cooke, I.D. (1986) Follicle growth patterns and endocrinological abnormalities in infertile women with minor degrees of endometriosis. *Br J Obstet Gynaecol* **93**, 852-8

44 Depot-medroxyprogesterone acetate (DMPA) Depo-Provera®:

A) Causes mammary tumours in beagle dogs.   TRUE
B) Is not licensed for use as a contraceptive in the USA.   FALSE
C) Is associated with a small increased risk of breast cancer in long-term users. FALSE
D) Is associated with an increased haemoglobin concentration in long-term users.   TRUE
E) May be associated with lower bone mineral density in long-term users.   TRUE

COMMENTS

Depot-medroxyprogesterone acetate (DMPA) is licensed in the UK for long-term use only in women in whom other contraceptives are contraindicated or unacceptable. After many years of controversy it was finally licensed for use in the USA in October 1992. The controversy arose mainly because of the finding that DMPA stimulated the growth of tumours of mammary tissue in beagle dogs (Anon. 1991). It is now widely recognised that the beagle dog is an inappropriate model for investigating the effects of steroid hormones in women. The World Health Organisation published a large multi-centre study which concluded that the risk of breast cancer was not increased in long-term users (WHO 1991). In the same year a group in New Zealand (Cundy *et al.* 1991) published the results of a small study which suggested that long term DMPA users had lower bone mineral density than controls. The study had some methodological flaws but raises the issue and suggests the need for further research

DMPA is a highly effective contraceptive which is of particular value in developing countries. The associated amenorrhoea in 40% of women and infrequent scanty periods in another 40% results in increased haemoglobin concentrations. There is some evidence to suggest that DMPA has a direct effect on erythropoietin.

REFERENCES

Anon. (1991) DMPA and breast cancer: the dog has had its day. *Lancet* **338**, 856-7

Cundy, T., Evans, M., Roberts, H. *et al.* (1991) Bone density in women receiving depot-medroxyprogesterone acetate for contraception. *BMJ* **303**, 13-16

WHO Collaborative Study of Neoplasia and Steroid Contraceptives (1991) Breast cancer and depot-medroxyprogesterone acetate: a multinational study. *Lancet* **338**, 833-8

45 With regard to patients receiving radical radiotherapy for carcinoma of the cervix, the following statements are correct:

A) The treatment-related mortality rate is greater than 1%.   FALSE

B) Late bowel complications most commonly occur within two years of completing treatment.   TRUE

C) Late bladder complications most commonly occur within one year of completing treatment.   FALSE

D) Treatment related complications are more common in the bladder than the bowel.   FALSE

E) The incidence of bowel complications is significantly increased by previous abdominal or pelvic surgery.   TRUE

COMMENTS

With modern methods the mortality rates for radical radiotherapy in cervical cancer are significantly less than 1%. Late morbidity of both small and large bowel, including perforation, is most common within the first two years after treatment. If the small bowel is immobilised by adhesions from previous surgery it may be damaged by the radiation. Large bowel complications include proctitis and rectal ulceration which usually settle with conservative management whilst stenosis and fistula formation require surgical intervention (Lanciano *et al.* 1992).

Late bladder morbidity is rare within the first year after therapy and most commonly occurs between two and three years after treatment. Frequency and dysuria caused by a sterile radiation cystitis, haematuria, ulceration and fistula formation are possible sequelae of radiotherapy for cervical cancer (Hamberger *et al.* 1983). Most authorities agree, however, that the bladder tolerates radiotherapy better than the bowel.

REFERENCES

Hamberger, A.D., Unal, A., Gershensen, D.M. *et al.* (1983) An analysis of severe complications of irradiation of carcinoma of the uterine cervix. *Int J Radiat Oncol Biol Phys* **9**, 367-71

Lanciano, R.M., Martz, K., Montana, G.S. *et al.* (1992) Influence of age, prior abdominal surgery, fraction size and dose on complications after radiation therapy for squamous cell cancer of the uterine cervix. *Cancer* **69**, 2124-30

46　A patient of 28 years presents with excessive hair growth involving the chin, upper lip, chest, areola, forearms and has a male escutcheon. Her height is 1.52 m and weight 82 kg (BMI = 36). She has a regular 30-day menstrual cycle. She finds the hair growth socially embarrassing and wishes treatment. The following statements can be made:

A) Hirsutism is commonly associated with adrenal hyperplasia.　　　　　　　FALSE
B) In obese patients with clinical polycystic ovarian disease (PCOD), the level of sex hormone binding globulin (SHBG) is increased.　　　　　　　　　　　　　FALSE
C) PCOD can occur in the presence of regular menstruation.　　　　　　　　TRUE
D) Dianette® functions by reducing production of SHBG and also by suppressing androgen production.　　　　　　　　　　　　　　　　　　　　　　　　　　FALSE
E) Deficiency of 21-hydroxylase can lead to androgen excess.　　　　　　　TRUE

COMMENTS

Hirsutism may be associated with PCOD but only rarely with adrenal hyperplasia or the androgen secreting tumours. The female production of androgens includes testosterone, androstenedione and dihydroepiandrostene. Testosterone is bound (in preference to oestrogen) to SHBG which is reduced in patients with PCOD. This is thought to be due to relative hyperinsulinaemia which allows more free testosterone to circulate (Weaver *et al.* 1989).

The spectrum of menstrual irregularity is great and ranges from a state of amenorrhoea to regular menses with a 28-day cycle. The diagnosis is made clinically from the phenotype and confirmed by either ultrasound of the ovaries, or biochemically, or both (Eden 1989).

Dianette® (Schering) is prescribed for the treatment of hirsutism. It combines ethynyl-oestradiol with cyproterone acetate. The latter acts as an anti-androgen due to its competitive inhibition of dihydrotestosterone binding to its receptor. The oestrogen component increases SHBG production and therefore lowers free testosterone levels in serum.

Steroid production in man is dependent upon enzyme reactions. 21-hydroxylase is necessary for the conversion of progesterone to deoxycortisone and also 17-alpha hydroxyprogesterone to deoxycortisol. The autosomal recessive disorder characterised by deficiency of 21-hydroxylase leads to excess androgen production – in particular androstenedione.

REFERENCES

Eden, J.A. (1989) The polycystic ovary syndrome. *Aust NZ J Obstet Gynaecol* **29**: 4, 403-16

Weaver, J.U., Noonan, K., Holly, J.M.P. *et al.* (1989) Decreased sex hormone binding globulin and insulin like growth factor binding protein in obesity. *J Endocrinol* **121** (Suppl), 254

47 **A healthy, 80-year-old woman presents with the symptoms of urgency, frequency, nocturia and incontinence. Her early management should include:**

A) An anterior colporrhaphy.	FALSE
B) Urethral pressure profilometry.	FALSE
C) A midstream specimen of urine for culture and sensitivities.	TRUE
D) Blood sugar estimation.	TRUE
E) Urethral dilatation.	FALSE

COMMENTS

Urinary problems are common in the elderly and often present with mixed symptoms. Although a urinary tract infection (UTI) may not be the sole cause, it will certainly exacerbate symptoms and urodynamic investigations, which require catheterisation, and will be uncomfortable in the presence of an infection. In addition, the results of the investigations may be inaccurate; so it is important to treat a UTI and repeat the midstream specimen of urine prior to further investigation. Diabetes mellitus may, of course, be an underlying cause for urinary frequency and urgency and should be excluded early.

Although urodynamic investigation, including cystometry and uroflowmetry, is very helpful in a case like this, urethral pressure profilometry is of no clinical relevance (Versi *et al.* 1986). The urethral pressure and length decrease with age and do not correlate with the clinical diagnosis at any age. Investigations should include a cystoscopy, to exclude bladder lesion such as transitional cell carcinoma which is relatively common in this age group, but urethral dilatation produces no long-term benefit unless there is proven urethral obstruction such as a stricture. In fact, repeated urethral dilatation may lead to incontinence or can cause stenosis of the urethra due to scarring from fibrosis.

An anterior colporrhaphy is a good operation for a cystocele – it is not the first line of treatment for incontinence or any urinary symptoms, especially prior to making an accurate diagnosis (Cardozo and Cutner 1992).

REFERENCES

Cardozo, L.D. and Cutner, A. (1992) Surgical management of genuine stress incontinence. *Contemp Rev Obstet Gynaecol* **4**, 36-41

Versi, E., Cardozo, L.D., Studd, J. *et al.* (1986) Evaluation of urethral pressure profilometry for the diagnosis of genuine stress incontinence. *World J Urology* **4**, 6-9

48   The following are the characteristic features of bacterial vaginosis:

A) There is drastic alteration in the normal vaginal flora with massive overgrowth of lactobacillus.   FALSE
B) Gardnerella is present.   TRUE
C) It produces a discharge of low pH <4.5.   FALSE
D) 'Clue cells' can be demonstrated on a wet mount of vaginal smear.   TRUE
E) It is uncommon in pregnancy.   FALSE

COMMENTS

Bacterial vaginosis is a frequent cause of vaginal discharge in women of the reproductive age group. The infection results from an imbalance in the vaginal flora with massive overgrowth of gardnerella and anaerobes (Eschenbach *et al.* 1989). Clinically an offensive, white, homogeneous adherent discharge of a high pH >5.0 is noted. Diagnosis is based on clinical findings and miscroscopic examination of wet mounts of vaginal discharge, when characteristic 'clue cells' (vaginal epithelial cells studded with coccobacilli obscuring the cell borders) can be demonstrated (Eschenbach *et al.* 1988). In pregnancy bacterial vaginosis has been implicated in premature rupture of membranes, premature labour, chorioamnionitis and puerperal pyrexia (Martius and Eschenbach 1990).

The antibiotic of choice for treatment of bacterial vaginosis is metronidazole 400 mg twice a day for seven days.

REFERENCES

Eschenbach, D.A., Hillier, S., Critchlow, C.M. *et al.* (1988) Diagnosis and clinical manifestations of bacterial vaginosis. *Am J Obstet Gynecol* **158**, 819-28

Eschenbach, D.A., Davick, P.R., Williams, B.L. *et al.* (1989) Prevalence of hydrogen peroxide producing lactobacillus species in normal women and women with bacterial vaginosis. *J Clin Microbiol* **27**: 2, 251-6

Martius, J. and Eschenbach, D.A. (1990) The role of bacterial vaginosis as a cause of amniotic fluid infection, chorioamnionitis and prematurity – a review. *Arch Gynecol Obstet* **247**, 1-13

49 A 52-year-old menopausal patient presents at clinic with menopausal symptoms and wishing advice about hormone replacement therapy (HRT). She is overweight at 80 kg, but is a non smoker. She has an insignificant past medical and surgical history but a family history suggestive of osteoporosis and her father died from a cerebrovascular accident at the age of 76. Which of the following statements are correct?

A) Orally administered oestrogens decrease low density lipoproteins (LDL).   TRUE

B) High density lipoproteins (HDL) have an inverse relationship with coronary heart disease.   TRUE

C) Oestrogens enhance bone resorption.   FALSE

D) The risk of endometrial carcinoma is not related to dose and duration of use of unopposed oestrogen.   FALSE

E) Transdermal HRT is more likely to affect patients with hypertension, cholelithiasis and hypercoagulable states.   FALSE

COMMENTS

It is estimated that 25-50% of the cardio-protective effect of orally administered oestrogens is related to an increase in the HDL fraction with reduction in LDL (Hazzard 1989). It is thought that lowering LDL is due to an increased apolipoprotein A synthesis and suppressed degradation of HDL particles due to inhibition of hepatic lipoprotein lipase (Schafer *et al.* 1983).

Oestrogens inhibit bone resorption. Other (non-hormonal) therapy can be used as an alternative and includes calcium, calcitonin and Vitamin D which permits increased calcium absorption. The bisphosphonates act in a similar way, reducing the number and effect of the osteoclasts in resorption. Recent studies have promoted this therapy to increase bone density in women with established vertebral fractures (Storm *et al.* 1990).

The risk of developing carcinoma of the endometrium is elevated after 2-4 years of use and continues to rise in a linear fashion thereafter. The risk returns to baseline after stopping treatment within two years (Whitehead *et al.* 1990). The tumours which do result appear to be less aggressive, with lower staging and also grading of disease.

Oral therapy passes directly through the liver and therefore affects production of hepatic proteins hepatically derived clotting factors VII, IX and X and theoretically renin substrate which may lead to increases in blood pressure. Non-oral routes do not have this effect (Cedars and Judd 1987).

REFERENCES

Cedars, M.I. and Judd, H.L. (1987) Non-oral routes of estrogen administration. *Obstet Gynecol Clin North Am* **14**, 269-98

Hazzard, W.R. (1989) Estrogen replacement and cardiovascular disease: serum lipids and blood pressure effects. *Am J Obstet Gynecol* **161**, 1847-53

Schafer, E.J., Foster, D.M. and Zech, L.A. (1983) Effects of estrogen administration on plasma lipoprotein metabolism in premenopausal females. *J Clin Endocrinol Metab* **57**, 262-7

Storm, T., Thamsborg, G., Steiniche, T. *et al.* (1990) Effect of intermittent cyclical etidronate therapy on bone mass and fracture rate in women with postmenopausal osteoporosis. *N Engl J Med* **322**, 1265-71

Whitehead, M.I., Hilliard, T.C. and Crook, D. (1990) The role and use of progestogens. *Obstet Gynecol* **75** (Suppl) 59-76

50 **A patient begins bleeding heavily one month after the evacuation of a hydatidiform mole. Ultrasound shows a transonic area in the uterine wall but no retained products in the cavity. The following treatments are worth considering to control the bleeding:**

A)	Methotrexate.	TRUE
B)	Oxytocic drugs.	FALSE
C)	Curettage.	FALSE
D)	Medroxyprogesterone acetate.	FALSE
E)	Uterine vessel ligation.	TRUE

COMMENTS

In this case, if there are persistently raised HCG levels, the diagnosis is invasive mole or choriocarcinoma. In either case, cancer chemotherapy usually is effective in reducing bleeding within a few days, probably arresting the invasive process.

Oxytocic drugs are effective haemostatic agents at the time of evacuation of a mole, but one month later they would be no more effective than in non-gestational cases of uterine bleeding. Curettage is only of value when there is retained molar tissue within the uterine cavity. Invasive disease cannot be eliminated by curettage which may result in further injury to the uterine wall. Progesterones have no reported favourable or unfavourable effect on gestational trophoblastic disease.

Hysterectomy may be life saving in cases of severe post-molar bleeding but there are a number of conservative measures which may preserve the uterus of a young woman. The transonic area may be an aneurysmal dilatation within the myometrium which is a relatively common implication of invasive mole. These arteriovenous malformations may be demonstrated by arteriography, and the bleeding may be controlled either by embolism or ligation of the feeding vessels (Belli *et al.* 1989).

REFERENCE

Belli, A-M., Hemingway, A.P., Neal, F.E. *et al.* (1989) Arterio-venous malformation of the uterus related to trophoblastic disease – a case for surgery or embolisation. *J Internat Radiol* **4**, 118-21

51 In postmenopausal women, bone loss:

A) Is reduced by exercise.   TRUE
B) Is reduced by calcium supplementation.   FALSE
C) Is increased by progestogens.   FALSE
D) Is accelerated by cigarette smoking.   TRUE
E) Is decreased by treatment with diphosphonates.   TRUE

COMMENTS

Osteoporosis and fractures are characteristic of the postmenopausal state. We are all aware of the beneficial effects of oestrogens in hormone replacement therapy, but other agents also play a part. Exercise (Brooks and Fahey 1985), treatment with diphosphonates (Storm *et al.* 1990) and calcitonin (Overgaard *et al.* 1989) have all been shown to reduce bone loss. Calcium supplementation is more controversial, but the weight of evidence suggests it is not effective. Progestogens may reduce bone loss, certainly they do not increase it, whereas cigarette smoking does.

REFERENCES

Brooks, G.A. and Fahey, T.D. (1985) 'Exercise physiology' in *Human Bioenergetics and its Applications*, pp. 343-4. New York: Macmillan

Overgaard, K., Riis, B.J., Christensen, C. *et al.* (1989) Nasal calcitonin for treatment of established osteoporosis. *Clin Endocrinol* **30**, 435-42

Storm, T., Thamsborg, G., Steiniche, E.T. *et al.* (1990) Effects of intermittent cyclical etidronate therapy on bone mass and fracture rate in women with postmenopausal osteoporosis. *N Engl J Med* **322** 1265-71

FURTHER READING

Purdie, D.C. (1991) The prevention of bone loss in women. *Curr Obstet Gynaecol* **1**: 1, 8-14

52 **In the presence of anti-phospholid antibodies (lupus anticoagulant and/or anticardiolipin antibodies), the following statements are correct:**

A) There may be a false-positive VDRL test. **TRUE**
B) There is a relationship with infertility. **TRUE**
C) Lupus anticoagulant may be demonstrated by prolongation of the activated partial thromboplastin time (APTT) not correctable by the addition of normal plasma or platelet neutralisation procedures. **FALSE**
D) There is proven relationship to unsuccessful pregnancy even in asymptomatic patients. **FALSE**
E) Thrombocytopaenia provides evidence of antiphospholipid antibody disease. **TRUE**

COMMENTS

Antiphospholipid antibodies such as lupus anticoagulant and anticardiolipin antibodies have been shown to be associated with a number of gynaecological and obstetric problems including infertility (Taylor *et al.* 1989), recurrent fetal loss (Lubbe and Liggings 1985), intrauterine growth retardation (Trippett 1989), endometriosis (Gleicher *et al.* 1987) and early onset pre-eclampsia.

The detection of antiphospholipid antibodies may be detected as a result of clinical evidence of antiphospholipid antibody syndrome (APAS) (such as arterial or venous thrombosis or thrombocytopaenia) (Harrison 1987); systemic lupus erythymatosis (SLE) or a false-positive VDRL. It is only in patients with SLE, APAS or lupus-like conditions that a definite relationship with pregnancy loss has been established (Out *et al.* 1991).

The diagnosis of lupus anticoagulant is dependent on the finding of an abnormally prolonged phospholipid dependent test of coagulation (e.g. APTT), kaolin clotting time (KCT) or dilute Russell viper venom time (dRVVT). The addition of normal plasma will not correct the coagulation, therefore indicating the presence of an inhibitor/anticoagulant. Confirmation that the coagulation defect is phospholipid dependent is then provided by the third step of the test by the addition of freeze-thawed platelets (platelet neutralisation procedure) which will reverse the prolongation of APTT (Trippett 1992).

REFERENCES

Gleicher, N., El Roeiy, Confino, E. *et al.* (1987) Is endometriosis an autoimmune disease? *Obstet Gynecol* **70**, 114-22

Harrison, E.N. (1987) Syndrome of the Black Swan. *Br J Rheumatol* **26**, 324-6

Lubbe, W.F. and Liggings, G.C. (1985) Lupus anticoagulant and pregnancy. *Am J Obstet Gynecol* **155**, 322-7

Out, H.J., Bruinse, H.W. and Derkson, R.H. (1991) Anti-phospholipid antibodies and pregnancy loss. *Hum Reprod* **6**, 6, 889-97

Taylor, P.V., Campbell, J.M. and Scott, J.S. (1989) Presence of autoantibodies in women with unexplained infertility. *Am J Obstet Gynecol* **161**, 377-9

Trippett, D.A. (1989) Antiphospholipid antibodies and recurrent pregnancy loss. *Am J Reprod Immunol* **20**, 52-67

Trippett, D.A. (1992) Obstetrical implications of antiphospholipid antibodies. *Baillière's Clin Obstet Gynaecol* **6**: 3, 507-18

53 Controlled ovarian hyperstimulation (COH) using gonadotrophin therapy is favoured by the majority of fertility clinics undertaking IVF because:

A)	COH results in a higher pregnancy rate compared with natural cycle IVF.	TRUE
B)	Timing of follicle aspiration is achieved by ultrasound assessment.	FALSE
C)	Multiple follicular development requires both FSH and LH.	FALSE
D)	Moderate–severe ovarian hyperstimulation syndrome is principally observed in presence of HCG.	TRUE
E)	HCG should be given for luteal support where GnRH analogues have been used prior to gonadotrophin ovarian stimulation.	FALSE

COMMENTS

In 1978 the first live birth was reported as a result of natural cycle *in vitro* fertilisation. Subsequently single and combination ovarian stimulation regimes were introduced which provided an increased number of oocytes. The use of human chorionic gonadotrophin (HCG) diminished problems associated with determining the start of the LH surge and enabled more accurate timing of follicle aspiration for oocyte retrieval. The net result was an increased pregnancy rate attributed to the transfer of more than a single embryo. Baird had shown in 1987 that the effect of elevating the FSH concentration above the threshold level early in the cycle is to stimulate the recruitment and development of first and second wave cohorts of follicles (Baird 1987).

Gonadotrophin therapy originally consisted of FSH and LH (HMG). Recently FSH alone has been shown to be capable of stimulating multiple follicular development. The advent of purer forms of FSH, e.g. Metrodin® HP and recombinant FSH may result in improved follicle growth and better quality embryos for transfer.

One of the major life-threatening complications of multiple follicular maturation is ovarian hyperstimulation syndrome (OHSS). Peripheral oestradiol concentration >2000 pg/ml associated with numerous medium-size follicles predisposes to moderate-severe ovarian hyperstimulation. HCG should be withheld as OHSS is principally observed in the presence of HCG whether exogenous or endogenous. Additional strategies have been described including transfer of embryos in a subsequent cycle and continuation of intranasal GnRH analogue. Recently Schoot and colleagues (1992) reported that proactive reduction of gonadotrophin stimulation allows smaller follicles to become atretic whilst sustaining the growth of larger follicles.

If GnRH analogues have been used prior to gonadotrophin ovarian stimulation, luteal support is required preferably in the form of progesterone, to avoid the undesirable effects of HCG stimulation.

REFERENCES

Baird, D.T. (1987) A model for follicular selection and ovulation: lessons from superovulation. *J Steroid Biochem* **27**, 15-23

Schoot, D.C., de Jong, F.H., Pache, D. *et al.* (1992) Growth patterns of ovarian follicles during the induction of ovulation with decreasing doses of human menopausal gonadotrophin following presumed selection in polycystic ovary syndrome. *Fertil Steril* **57**: 5, 1117-20

FURTHER READING

Steptoe, P.C., Edwards, P.G. and Walters, D.E. (1986) Observation on 767 clinical pregnancies and 500 births after human *in vitro* fertilisation. *Human Reprod* **1**, 89-94

54 The following statements about intrauterine contraceptive devices (IUCDs) are correct:

A) It is accepted by WHO that all copper IUCDs have similar efficacy, with no important differences in efficacy as duration of use increases. FALSE

B) Excluding episodes in the first 20 days after insertion, there is now good evidence that there is no IUCD-related excess risk of pelvic inflammatory disease (PID) and no increase in risk with long-term use. TRUE

C) Two follow-up visits after IUCD insertion are now recommended, one at around two weeks and the other at six-eight weeks. TRUE

D) Among symptomless IUCD users with cervical cytology showing Actinomyces-like organisms (ALOs), simple removal of the device without antibiotics leads to negative findings in follow-up smears. TRUE

E) It is unnecessary to change any copper IUCD fitted above the age of 40, and the same device may be left *in situ* until contraception is no longer required following the menopause. TRUE

COMMENTS

Good multi-centre comparisons of current copper devices, by WHO and the Population Council, have established clear differences in the efficacy of different designs (World Health Organisation 1987). In particular, the Nova T®/Novagard® has a significantly higher failure rate than the T-shaped devices bearing copper bands on their transverse arms – represented in the UK by the Ortho Gyne-T® Cu-380 Slimline. In the WHO studies the Nova-T® had a failure rate of between one and two per 100 women at one year whereas the banded devices gave estimates well below one. In a Population Council Study (Sivin *et al.* 1991), the annual failure rate in the first two years was 0.4 per 100 woman years, dropping after two years to 0.2 and zero from Year five through to Year seven. The cumulative failure rate to seven years was only 1.4 per 100 women. These studies imply no less effectiveness than the COC and form the basis for the official recommendation of the US Food and Drug Administration, also accepted by authorities in the UK, that the banded (Cu-380 type) IUCD should normally remain *in situ* for at least eight years.

Support for the answers to (B) and (C) comes from analysis by WHO of a large data base; nearly 23 000 IUCD insertions with over 51 000 woman years of follow up, based on multi-centre comparative studies from 23 countries representing every continent of the world (Farley *et al.* 1992):

> PID risk was more than six times higher during the 20 days after insertion than during later times (unadjusted rates 9.7 versus 1.4 per 1000 woman years respectively); the risk was low and constant for up to eight years of follow up. Rates varied according to geographical area and were inversely associated with age . . . our findings indicate that PID among IUCD users is most strongly related to the insertion process and a background risk of sexually transmissible disease.

Coupled with the lack of any change in the incidence rate after the first 20 days (i.e. no duration-of-use effect) the fact that there was not a single case of PID among 4301 IUCD users in China (where the background risk of STDs and PID was low) is strong confirmation that IUCD use *per se* does not increase the risk of PID above background.

The WHO finding of a seven-fold increased risk of PID in the 20 days after insertion requires comment and should affect practice. It is not necessarily caused by poor IUCD insertion technique. It is consistent with the demonstration of transient microbiological contamination of the uterine cavity following insertion (Mishell 1966). STD organisms being carried asymptomatically in the cervix may be transferred by the insertion process to the uterus and tubes.

In most societies screening for STDs, particularly *Chlamydia trachomatis* (Fish *et al.* 1987), should ideally be performed before IUCDs are inserted or reinserted. One study of prophylactic antibiotics showed a reduced risk of infection after insertion, but the difference was not statistically significant (Sinei *et al.* 1990). After appropriate screening, therefore, it may be more advantageous to arrange a follow-up contact or visit at either one or two weeks post-insertion – with vigorous treatment (probably including device removal) in those cases with PID symptoms and signs. A further early follow-up visit at six-eight weeks (as currently practised) is also advisable, to detect and manage other problems such as partial and complete expulsions which are more common in the early weeks.

Mao and Guillebaud (1984) showed that IUCD removal without antibiotics led in all cases to smears negative for ALO carriage when repeated 6–12 months after the initial visit; and this was significantly different to the rate of persistence of the cytology findings in similarly asymptomatic women whose devices were left *in situ*. Complete clearance of the ALO finding was also noted in seven women who had a copper IUCD immediately reinserted at the time of removal. Singh *et al.* (1989) in a larger series of 100 asymptomatic women confirmed the main finding, that simple IUCD removal led to 100% clearance of ALOs on subsequent cytology, without use of antibiotics. After discussion with the woman, removal of the device (and its immediate replacement with a new one if desired) therefore is the nub of the recommendations of the National Association of Family Planning Doctors (1991). Singh takes a different view, in that if a patient is symptom-free the IUCD can be left in place and the smear simply repeated in six months, with treatment if symptoms develop. Unless the woman chooses that course the NAFPD policy is preferable, because of the difficulty of ensuring 100% follow-up and the impossibility of predicting which woman might have the rare but catastrophic sequelae of pelvic actinomycosis. It is clear that antibiotics are unnecessary in the absence of symptoms of PID on positive results for Actinomyces culture from the laboratory; but in the latter event a penicillin is required for at least 90 days.

Most studies show that pregnancy rates with copper IUCDs do not increase or decline with increasing duration of use. This is partly because of declining fertility with increasing age. The UK FPA and NAFPD issued a joint statement (Newton and Tacchi 1990) that all currently marketed copper devices may be left *in situ* for five years – now increased to eight years for the T-Cu-380 (see above). In a subsequent letter to the *Lancet* (Tacchi 1990), it was also stated as policy that any copper device fitted above the age of 40 may continue *in situ* until the menopause. This judgement was based on the known risks of reinsertion (including infection, see above) as compared with the strengthened efficacy of any copper IUCD above the age of 40, due to declining fertility.

REFERENCES

Farley, T.M., Rosenberg, M.J., Rowe, P.J. *et al.* (1992) Intrauterine devices and pelvic inflammatory disease: an international perspective. *Lancet* **339**, 785-8

Fish, A.N., Robinson, G.E., Bounds, W. *et al.* (1987) *Chlamydia trachomatis* in various groups of contraceptors: preliminary observations. *Br J Fam Plann* **13**, 84-7

Mao, K. and Guillebaud, J. (1984) Influence of removal of intrauterine contraceptive devices on colonisation of the cervix by Actinomyces-like organisms. *Contraception* **30**, 535-44

Mishell, D.R. (1966) The intrauterine device: a bacteriologic study of the endometrial cavity. *Am J Obstet Gynecol* **96**, 119-26

National Association of Family Planning Doctors (1991) Report of the Clinical Scientific and Advisory Committee. *Br J Fam Plann* **16**, 152

Newton, J. and Tacchi, D. (1990) Long-term use of copper intrauterine devices. *Lancet* **335**, 1322-3

Sinei, S.K., Schulz, K.F. and Lamptey, P.R. (1990) Preventing IUCD-related pelvic infection: the efficacy of prophylactic doxycycline at insertion. *Br J Obstet Gynaecol* **97**, 412-19

Singh, M.M., Ingham, H.R., Wadehra, V. *et al.* (1989) Endometrial culture in IUD users with actinomycosis-like organisms (ALOs) on cervical smears. *Br J Fam Plann* **15**, 3-6

Sivin, I., Stern, J., Coutinho, E. *et al.* (1991) Prolonged intrauterine contraception: a seven-year randomized study of the levonorgestrel 28 mcg per day (LNg 20) and the copper T380 Ag IUDs. *Contraception* **44**, 473-80

Tacchi, D. (1990) Long-term use of copper intrauterine devices. *Lancet* **336**, 182

World Health Organisation (1987) Mechanism of action, safety and efficacy of intrauterine devices. *Technical Report Series* **753**. Geneva: WHO

55 Leiomyosarcoma of the uterus:

A) Is more common in black women.   TRUE
B) Carries a better prognosis in premenopausal women.   TRUE
C) Responds well to radiotherapy.   FALSE
D) Accounts for 5% of uterine malignancies.   FALSE
E) Carries a universally poor prognosis.   FALSE

COMMENTS

Leiomyosarcoma of the uterus is more common in black women than Caucasians, possibly because of the higher incidence of benign myomas, and tends to carry a worse prognosis in this group (Christopherson et al. 1972). The prognosis tends to be better in younger patients. Unfortunately, there is no effective adjuvant therapy in this condition following initial surgery. The incidence of uterine sarcomas is around 5% of all uterine malignancies and in most series leiomyosarcomas account for about 40% of sarcomas (Lurian and Piver 1992). The most important prognostic factor in leiomyosarcomas is the number of mitotic figures seen per ten high-power fields. If less than five are detected, the prognosis is excellent.

REFERENCES

Christopherson, W.M., Williamson, E.O. and Gray, L.A. (1972) Leiomyosarcoma of the uterus. *Cancer* **29**, 1512-17

Lurian, J.R. and Piver, M.S. (1992) 'Uterine sarcomas: clinical features and management' in M. Coppleson, J.M. Monaghan, P. Morrow and M.H. Tattersall (Eds) *Gynecologic Oncology*, pp. l27-42. Edinburgh: Churchill Livingstone

56   With regard to endometriosis and symptomology, which of the following statements are correct?

A) Congestive dysmenorrhoea, deep dyspareunia and pelvic pain are the most common symptoms associated with mild endometriosis.   TRUE

B) The severity of pelvic pain reflects the extent of pelvic endometriosis.   FALSE

C) About 70% of women with chronic pelvic pain will have laparoscopically documented pelvic endometriosis.   FALSE

D) LHRH analogues are superior to danazol with respect to menstrual symptoms relief.   FALSE

E) LHRH analogues (A) are more effective than other medical treatments in preventing a recurrence of symptomatic pelvic endometriosis.   FALSE

COMMENTS

The majority of women with endometriosis usually complain of congestive dysmenorrhoea, pelvic discomfort and dyspareunia (Chatman and Ward 1982; Jansen and Russel 1986). It is believed that some women with minimal endometriosis complain of severe pain and conversely women with extensive disease may exhibit little or no discomfort (Ranney 1980). A prospective questionnaire-based study, involving 1200 premenopausal women (Mahmood et al. 1991) did not substantiate the above belief.

The pathophysiology of chronic pelvic pain is poorly understood (Messer 1992). The published data are inconsistent, varying between 4 and 65%, averaging around 25% (Mahmood and Templeton 1991).

Several open randomised or double-blind placebo studies have compared the efficacy of GnRH agonists with danazol. Side-effects associated with GnRH agonists are mainly related to the hypo-oestrogenic state. The most troublesome side-effects of danazol are related to the androgenicity of the drug. However, none of the comparative trials have shown significant differences between any of the GnRH agonists investigated and danazol with respect to symptom relief or impact on disease (Shaw 1992).

The natural history of endometriosis is poorly understood (Mahmood and Templeton 1990). Spontaneous regression has been described in mild cases. In general, regression of endometriotic implants is seen in between 50% and 90% of patients. Up to 15% of patients show active progression on treatment. Adhesions and large ovarian endometriomas do not respond. Up to 50% of patients have symptomatic recurrence by five years. There are no data described confirming the superiority of LHRH-A for long-term benefits (Shaw 1992).

REFERENCES

Chatman, D.L. and Ward, A.B. (1982) Endometriosis in adolescents. *J Reprod Med* **27**, 156-60

Jansen, R.P.S. and Russel, P. (1986) Non-pigmented endometriosis: clinical laparoscopic and pathologic definition. *Am J Obstet Gynecol* **155**, 1154-9

Mahmood, T.A. and Templeton, A. (1990) The impact of treatment on the natural history of endometriosis. *Hum Reprod* **5**, 956-70

Mahmood, T.A. and Templeton, A. (1991) Prevalence and genesis of endometriosis. *Hum Reprod* **6**, 544-9

Mahmood, T.A., Templeton, A., Thomson, L. *et al.* (1991) Menstrual symptomatology among women with pelvic endometriosis. *Br J Obstet Gynaecol* **98**, 558-63

Messer, R.H. (1992) Chronic pelvic pain. *Curr Opin Obstet Gynecol* **4**, 6, 886-90

Ranney, B. (1980) Endometriosis: pathogenesis, symptoms and findings. *Clin Obstet Gynaecol* **23**, 865-70

Shaw, R.W. (1992) Treatment of endometriosis. *Lancet* **340**, 1267-71

57   Between 80% and 90% of couples attempting to conceive are successful after one year. The following statements are correct:

A) Tubal damage accounts for 14% of all causes of infertility.	TRUE
B) Resources currently devoted to tubal surgery for severe disease could be more efficiently used if reallocated to assisted conception techniques.	TRUE
C) Reversal of female sterilisation is not effective.	FALSE
D) Diagnosis of tubal damage is best made by laparoscopy alone.	FALSE
E) The ectopic pregnancy rate following surgery for distal tubal occlusion is 23%.	TRUE

COMMENTS

The 'unexplained' group of infertility problems accounts for approximately 30% of all those couples failing to conceive after two years, although further specific investigations of sperm and ovum function may yet identify causes in these couples (Haxton and Black 1987; Hull *et al.* 1985). Tubal damage alone is a cause of infertility in 14% and ovulatory failure in 27%. Other proportions are male factor 19% and endometriosis 5%.

The success of surgery for tubal damage is greater in those with mild pathology than in those with severe damage and a decision on treatment should only be made after careful evaluation by laparoscopy and hysterosalpingography (Winston and Margara 1991). Mild pathology in which no adhesions exist is associated with a far higher pregnancy rate than if the damage is severe and the tubes are occluded at the distal end (Singhal *et al.* 1991). Reversal of sterilisation on the other hand carries a far better prognosis and birth rates greater than 50% are commonly achieved. The method and site of tubal occlusion is, however, relevant to the success (Yue and Fa 1989).

Tubal surgery should not be undertaken without clear indication that the damage is not severe. Selection should be made using both laparoscopy and hysterosalpingography (Winston and Margara 1991). Where the damage is severe or where there is not the expertise for microtubal surgery, better results may be achieved by assisted conception techniques. A pregnancy rate of 18% and a maternity rate of 13% per cycle of treatment should be achieved for couples where tubal damage is the sole cause of infertility (HFEA 1992).

The most common site for tubal obstruction is the distal end and, depending upon severity, pregnancy rates of 6-30% may be achieved. The ectopic rate, however, is approximately one quarter of these. The ectopic rate in the general population is about 0.8% (Lavy *et al.* 1987).

REFERENCES

Haxton, M.J. and Black, W.P. (1987) The aetiology of infertility in 1162 investigated couples. *Clin Exp Obstet Gynecol* **14**, 75-9

Hull, M.G., Glazener, C.M., Kelly, M.J. *et al.* (1985) Population study of the causes, treatment and outcome of infertility. *BMJ* **291**, 1693-7

HFEA (1992) *Annual Report of the Human Fertilisation and Embryology Authority*. London: HMSO

Lavy, G., Diamond, M.P. and DeCherney, A.H. (1987) Ectopic pregnancy: its relationship to tubal reconstructive surgery. *Fertil Steril* **47**, 543-56

Singhal, V., Li, T.C. and Cooke, I.D. (1991) An analysis of factors influencing the outcome of 232 consecutive tubal microsurgery cases. *Br J Obstet Gynaecol* **98**, 7, 628-36

Winston, R.M. and Margara, R.A. (1991) Microsurgical salpingostomy is not an obsolete procedure. *Br J Obstet Gynaecol* **98**, 637-42

Yue, P. and Fa, Y. (1989) Microsurgical reversal of female sterilisation. *J Reprod Med* **34**, 451-5

58 A 21-year-old woman comes to see you because she is embarrassed by bed wetting. Although she became dry at the normal age, she started wetting the bed again when she was in her teens and none of the remedies which her local doctor has tried have helped. Recently she started living with her boyfriend and is taking the combined oral contraceptive pill. She is relatively free of symptoms during the day but sometimes loses urine when she has an orgasm. Which of the following statements are correct?

A)	It is likely that she has voiding difficulties, with a persistent urinary residual.	FALSE
B)	Her symptoms may be exacerbated by the combined oral contraceptive pill.	FALSE
C)	The most likely urodynamic abnormality would be detrusor instability.	TRUE
D)	She should be given imipramine 5 mg *nocte*.	FALSE
E)	DDAVP® (desmopressin) is likely to be helpful.	TRUE

COMMENTS

Nocturnal enuresis, in adults, is not uncommon and may restart even after a child has been dry for a number of years. It is not related to taking the combined oral contraceptive pill.

When nocturnal enuresis is the only symptom, quite often there are no urodynamic abnormalities, although detrusor instability may be the underlying cause (Mayo and Burns 1990). However, coital incontinence which occurs at the time of orgasm is associated with detrusor instability, making this the most likely urodynamic abnormality in this case (Hilton 1988). It is worth carrying out a urodynamic assessment as this may help the patient to understand her problem and will also avoid the use of inappropriate drugs.

Imipramine may be useful for both the bed-wetting and the incontinence at orgasm but should be given in a dose of about 50 mg *nocte* in order to be effective (Castleden *et al.* 1981). Nowadays the most popular treatment is DDAVP® (desmopressin), which is a synthetic analogue of vasopressin (Hilton and Stanton 1982). It is given as a nasal spray or snuff (20-40 mg *nocte*), although it will soon be available in tablet form. DDAVP® is very effective treatment for bed-wetting and has been shown to be safe for long-term use if taken only once in a 24-hour period (Carter *et al.* 1992). It cannot be used in elderly people with heart disease or hypertension.

REFERENCES

Carter, P.G., McConnell, A.A., Abrams, P. (1992) The safety and efficacy of DDAVP® in the elderly. *Neurol Urodyn* **11**: 4, 421-42

Castelden, C.M., George, C.F., Renwick, A.G. *et al.* (1981) Imipramine – a possible alternative to current therapy for urinary incontinence in the elderly. *J Urol* **125**, 318-20

Hilton, P. (1988) Urinary incontinence during sexual intercourse: a common but rarely volunteered symptom. *Br J Obstet Gynaecol* **95**, 377-81

Hilton, P. and Stanton, S.L. (1982) The use of desmopressin (DDAVP®) in nocturnal urine frequency in the female. *Br J Urol* **54**, 252-5

Mayo, M.E. and Burns, M.W. (1990) Urodynamic studies in children who wet. *Br J Urol* **65**: 6, 641-5

59 **With regard to *Chlamydia trachomatis*, which of the following are correct?**

A) It is an important cause of pelvic infection following first-trimester termination of pregnancy.   TRUE

B) It can be detected in approximately 20% of women requesting termination of pregnancy.   FALSE

C) It can be effectively treated by erythromycin 500 mg b.d. given for 48 hours before termination of pregnancy.   FALSE

D) Its eradication should be checked by repeat screening two weeks after treatment.   FALSE

E) There is a strong association between the presence of *C. trachomatis* and gonococcus in endocervical samples.   FALSE

COMMENTS

If *C. trachomatis* is detected prior to the procedure, 20–25% of women will develop post-abortion pelvic infection. Most UK studies from clinics providing termination of pregnancy have reported infection in 8–10% of women requesting this procedure. If time allows it is better to give a full ten-day course of treatment with erythromycin 500 mg four times a day before the procedure is carried out.

There is some uncertainty as to the optimum time to allow after treatment is completed before checking for eradication. Between four and six weeks is probably necessary and advice should be given to use condoms to avoid reinfection together with screening and treatment of sexual partners. There is no association with gonococcal infection.

APPROPRIATE READING

Qvigstad, E. (1983) Pelvic inflammatory disease associated with *C. trachomatis* after therapeutic abortion. *Br J Ven Dis* **59**, 189-92

Cohn, M. and Stewart, P. (1992) Prevalence of potential pathogens in cervical canal before termination of pregnancy. *BMJ* **304**, 1479

60 The following conditions are absolute contraindications to oestrogen-containing hormone replacement therapy (HRT):

A) Hypertension.   FALSE
B) Ischaemic heart disease.   FALSE
C) Deep vein thrombosis (DVT).   FALSE
D) Endometrial cancer.   FALSE
E) Breast cancer.   TRUE

COMMENTS

The potential dangers of HRT have been extrapolated from the effects observed with the oral contraceptive pill. Synthetic oestrogens contained within oral contraceptives are responsible for a degree of hypertension but in population-based studies HRT has been shown to cause a fall in mean blood pressure (Nachtigall *et al.* 1979). A small number of women may show a substantial increase (Wren 1988).

It is well established that the effect of exogenous oestrogen therapy on plasma lipids is to raise HDL cholesterol (Bush and Miller 1987) and therefore it should and does reduce the incidence of ischaemic heart disease in postmenopausal women (Ross *et al.* 1981). Although progestogens may counteract this effect, there is no contraindication to therapy unless the woman has other risk factors such as oestrogen-sensitive hypertension.

The incidence of DVT is also more common in women using combined oral contraception but it has not shown to be more common in women using HRT (Boston Collaborative Drug Surveillance Program 1974), presumably because although these hormones increase hepatic protein synthesis there is little effect on clotting factors.

Although both endometrial and breast cancer are hormone dependent, the survival of women with early-stage and apparently completely resected endometrial cancer has been shown not to be adversely affected by exogenous oestrogen therapy (Creasman *et al.* 1986). There have been no such studies in breast cancer which in general is a more aggressive tumour and its presence should be regarded as the only absolute contraindication.

REFERENCES

Boston Collaborative Drug Surveillance Program (1974) Surgically confirmed gallbladder disease, venous thrombo-embolism and breast tumors in relation to postmenopausal estrogen therapy. *N Engl J Med* **290**, 15-19

Bush, T.L. and Miller, V.T. (1987) 'Effects of pharmacologic agents used during menopause impacts on lipids and lipoproteins' in D.R. Mishell (Ed.) *Menopause: Physiology and Pharmacology*, pp. 187-208. Chicago; London: Year Book Medical Publishers

Creasman, W.T., Henderson, D., Hinshaw, W. *et al.* (1986) Estrogen replacement therapy in the patient treated for endometrial cancer. *Obstet Gynecol* **67**, 326-30

Nachtigall, L.E., Nachtigall, R.H., Nachtigall, R.D. *et al.* (1979) Estrogen replacement therapy 11. A prospective relationship to carcinoma, cardiovascular and metabolic disorders. *Obstet Gynecol* **54**, 74-9

Ross, R.K., Paganini-Hill, A., Mack, T.M. *et al.* (1981) Menopausal oestrogen therapy and protection from death from ischaemic heart disease. *Lancet* **1** (8225): 858-60

Wren, B.G. (1988) 'Hypertension and thrombosis with postmenopausal oestrogen therapy' in J.W.W. Studd and M.I. Whitehead (Eds.) *The Menopause*, pp. 181-9. Oxford: Blackwell Scientific

61 A woman aged 36 years attended a gynaecology OPD in an NHS Trust Hospital with a request for sterilisation. She was seen by a registrar who talked to her about the procedure but did not record their conversation in the notes. The patient then signed a consent form which included the clause:

After this procedure I am aware that I may not become or remain infertile.

Laparoscopic sterilisation was performed two months later by a senior registrar using clips to occlude the fallopian tubes. Six months later the patient found she was pregnant. Pregnancy termination at 10 weeks' gestation was offered but declined, and she gave birth to a healthy son. At the subsequent re-sterilisation it was found that on one side of the pelvis the clip was on the round ligament. The patient decided to take legal action, claiming that the operation was performed negligently and that she had not been told of the risk of failure. The advice given to the defendant is likely to be:

A) That pre-operative counselling about the risk of failure will be considered adequate.	FALSE
B) That as the consent form acknowledged the risk of failure there was no liability for such a failure.	FALSE
C) That the senior registrar was liable for the operation failure.	FALSE
D) That the consultant was liable for the operation failure.	FALSE
E) That damages awarded could include the cost of bringing up the child.	TRUE

COMMENTS

According to James (1991) failed sterilisation is the most common subject for litigation in gynaecology, comprising 25% of all claims notified. Proper preoperative counselling must be given and documented. In her article on risk management, James writes:

> A record of the counselling given should be made in the patient's case notes. The absence of a contemporary note may make a claim difficult to defend even if it is the doctor's stated practice to advise all patients that sterilization has a failure rate, since the patient's account of events is likely to be preferred. It would be argued that the patient's recollection is based on a single personal experience whereas the doctor may have departed from his usual practice on that particular occasion for a number of different reasons.

Failures of sterilisation techniques can be divided into two groups: method failures and operator failures. Method failures are those cases where the technique has been properly performed on the correct structure, that is, the fallopian tube. Borten (1986) gives the expected rate of method failure as between 0.9 and 0.6 per thousand, with the lowest rate obtained with the use of diathermy, the highest rate with the use of spring-loaded clips and an intermediate rate of silastic bands.

Operator failure is probably more common. The reasons include misidentification of pelvic structures and inadequate technique, and clearly represent unacceptable practice. Care must also be taken to advise all patients of the risk of a luteal phase pregnancy being present at the time of sterilisation.

As the hospital concerned is an NHS Trust this accident will have happened after 1990 and hence the system of Crown Indemnity is in force. With regards to litigation the health authorities and NHS Trusts are exclusively liable for the negligence of doctors in their hospitals. Prior to 1990 doctors were separately liable and whether or not the consultant would have then been responsible for the actions of his juniors would depend on the perception of their level of competence. By virtue of his position the senior registrar should have been competent to perform this procedure; in *Rosen v Edgar* [1986] (reported in Nelson-Jones and Burton 1990) it was ruled that a consultant was not liable for the actions of a senior registrar although that doctor was junior to him and answerable to him for his actions.

Although the patient was offered a pregnancy termination her refusal to accept this would not have altered or reduced the defendant's liability. In 1985 the Court of Appeal held in a case of failed sterilisation with a plaintiff who had already undergone one abortion:

. . . that the Plaintiff's refusal to undergo an abortion was not so unreasonable as to eclipse the surgeon's negligence. Save in the most exceptional circumstances the Court should not declare it unreasonable for a woman to decline to have an abortion in a case where there is no evidence that there were any medical or psychiatric grounds for terminating the particular pregnancy. Consequently the defendant's plea of *novus actus interveniens* failed, as did their argument that the Plaintiff had failed to take reasonable steps to minimise the damage.

. . . that it is not contrary to public policy to recover damages for the birth of a child, whether healthy or abnormal.

REFERENCES

Borten, M. (1986) *Laparoscopic Complication, Prevention and Management*, pp. 383-90. Toronto: B.C. Decker

James, C. (1991) Risk management in obstetrics and gynaecology. *J Med Defence Union* 7, 36-8

Nelson-Jones, R. and Burton, F. (1990) *Medical Negligence Case Law*, pp. 205-6; 302-3. London: Format Publishing

FURTHER READING

Lewis, C.J. (1992) *Medical Negligence: A Practical Guide* (2nd ed.). Croydon: Tolley Publishing

62 A 56-year-old woman who has breast cancer has been on tamoxifen for five years. She presents to the gynaecology OPD with postmenopausal bleeding and is found on examination to have an enlarged uterus. Which of the following statements are correct?

A) This is unlikely to be endometrial cancer as the two cancers rarely occur together. FALSE
B) Tamoxifen is unlikely to be causative as it produces endometrial atrophy. FALSE
C) Tamoxifen's efficacy in breast cancer is related only to its anti-oestrogenic properties. FALSE
D) The uterine enlargement is unlikely to be due to fibroids as these would have shrunk in a patient on tamoxifen. FALSE
E) An ultrasound scan estimating endometrial thickness of 7 mm would suggest endometrial carcinoma in this patient. FALSE

COMMENTS

Tamoxifen is an enigmatic drug. It was initially thought to be an anti-oestrogen in humans but it has become apparent that it has many oestrogenic properties. It causes endometrial hyperplasia in a majority of women although not all of these will have associated menstrual problems. In fact, some note an improvement (Lumsden *et al.* 1989a).

An endometrial thickness of 7 mm would be highly suggestive of endometrial carcinoma in women not on this drug. Tamoxifen appears to bind to oestrogen receptors in the uterus (Lumsden *et al.* 1989b) and due to its partial agonist action, fibroids either stay the same size or enlarge. It has even been demonstrated that it may have agonist actions on the breast which would suggest that its efficacy in breast cancer may result in part from other mechanisms. These alternative mechanisms may help explain why it is effective in oestrogen-receptor negative disease.

REFERENCES

Lumsden, M.A., West, C.P., Hillier, H. *et al.* (1989a) Estrogenic action of tamoxifen in women treated with luteinizing hormone releasing hormone agonist (goserelin) – lack of shrinkage of uterine fibroids. *Fertil Steril* **52**, 6, 924-9

Lumsden, M.A., West, C.P., Hawkins, R.A. *et al.* (1989b) The binding of steroids to myometrium and leiomyomata (fibroids) in women treated with the gonadotrophin-releasing agonist Zoladex (ICI 118630). *J Endocrinol* **121**, 389-96

63   The following statements about potential drug interactions with oral contraception are correct:

A) A user of Femulen® (ethynodiol diacetate) who is prescribed a five-day course of tetracycline should be instructed to take additional contraceptive precautions.   FALSE

B) If a woman has been taking a broad spectrum antibiotic such as tetracycline long term (or any time in excess of two weeks) before the combined pill is prescribed, there is no need to advise extra contraceptive precautions.   TRUE

C) The COC cannot be fully relied upon using a standard treatment regimen if there is co-treatment with any of the following: co-trimoxazole, sodium valproate, clonazepam, vigabatrin, lamotrigine.   FALSE

D) A triphasic pill would not be a good contraceptive choice for a woman treated with carbamazepine (Tegretol®).   TRUE

E) If a stronger COC regimen has been used during therapy with a recognised enzyme inducer, once the drug is discontinued there can be immediate return to a normal low-dose COC.   FALSE

COMMENTS

Femulen® is a progestogen-only pill and as such its bioavailability is unaffected by antibiotics. Enterohepatic recirculation of ethinyl oestradiol is due to large bowel flora which are capable of hydrolysing the liver conjugates, followed by reabsorption of unchanged oestrogen into the portal circulation (Back and Orme 1990). The artificial progestogens are not similarly recycled, hence any antibiotics altering this flora can only lower the blood levels of ethinyl oestradiol (and then only in an unknown small minority of women).

Even with the combined pill the small risk of a breakthrough pregnancy is not believed to continue beyond about two weeks' use of the antibiotic (Back and Orme 1990), due to the development by the relevant flora of antibiotic resistance within that timescale. Therefore the advice to current users of the COC or the similar Dianette® – which is to use additional contraceptive precautions for the duration of any antibiotic treatment and for seven days thereafter (with omission of the next pill-free interval if the last seven tablets are involved) – does not apply if, or after, such courses have lasted more than 14 days.

None of the drugs listed at (C) are enzyme inducers. Indeed, co-trimoxazole (probably by virtue of its sulphonamide component) acts as a mild liver enzyme inhibitor, therefore if anything increasing the contraceptive efficacy of the COC (Grimmer et al. 1983).

Triphasic pills are entirely unsuitable for use with carbamazepine since they are in general among the lowest dose compounds available. Since the interacting drug makes the metabolising liver enzymes more active, a stronger formulation is recommended. It is usual to start with a 50 µg oestrogen compound, but to be prepared if breakthrough bleeding occurs (this being a marker of low blood levels) to give additional tablets, to a maximum of 100 µg of oestrogen daily. Since the pill-free interval is the time during which ovarian activity may return (Guillebaud 1987), it obviously increases the efficacy of the method if these pill-free times are eliminated/shortened. Therefore, current accepted practice is to use a monophasic COC, but to give it by the so-called tricycle regimen – three packets in a row followed by a pill-free interval, which is ideally also shortened to four rather than the usual seven days. The efficacy of the method is greatly increased by thus having fewer and shorter contraceptively-dangerous, pill-free intervals. This regimen is also indicated for any woman who has suffered a previous 'breakthrough' conception (Guillebaud 1989).

Once liver enzyme induction is established, it can take a considerable time for the enzyme activity to return to normal. It is therefore advised that when relevant antiepileptic drugs are discontinued (barbiturates, carbamazepine, phenytoin, primidone, also griseofulvin and spironolactone), there is no return to a standard low-dose regimen for at least four weeks, and eight weeks after long-term barbiturate use. Rifampicin is so powerful that after as little as two days' use there should be no reliance on a standard COC regimen for the subsequent four weeks (Orme and Back 1991).

REFERENCES

Back, D.J. and Orme, M.L. (1990) Pharmacokinetic drug interactions with oral contraceptives. *Clin Pharmacokinet* **18**, 472-84

Grimmer, S.F., Allen, W.L., Back, D.J. *et al.* (1983). The effect of co-trimoxazole on oral contraceptive steroids in women. *Contraception* **28**, 53-9

Guillebaud, J. (1987) The forgotten pill – and the paramount importance of the pill-free week. *Br J Fam Plann* **12** (suppl), 35-43

Guillebaud, J. (1989) 'Practical prescribing of the combined oral contraceptive pill' in M. Filshie and J. Guillebaud (Eds) *Contraception: Science and Practice*, pp. 76-82. London: Butterworth Heinemann

Orme, M. and Back, D.J. (1991) Oral contraceptive steroids – pharmacological issues of interest to the prescribing physician. *Adv Contr* **7**, 325-31

64 At around the time of the menopause:

A) Vasomotor symptoms may commence before menstruation has ceased. TRUE

B) The incidence of depression is no more common than in the reproductive era of life. FALSE

C) Disturbed sleep patterns are helped by hormone replacement therapy (HRT). TRUE

D) The use of progestogens is necessary if topical conjugated equine oestrogen cream is used for the treatment of vaginal dryness in a woman with a uterus. FALSE *True*

E) Ischaemic heart disease is more common in women with an earlier menopause. TRUE

COMMENTS

Ovarian function begins to decline in the mid-thirties. Oestrogen levels may begin to fall some time after and give rise to menopausal symptoms whilst oestrogen levels are still sufficient to cause menstruation (Bungay *et al.* 1980).

Although there is no evidence that declining ovarian function is responsible, there is a definite increase in the incidence of minor psychological symptoms such as depression in a cohort of women of approximately 50 years of age (Bungay *et al.* 1980) and in postmenopausal women when compared to their premenopausal counterparts (Hunter *et al.* 1986).

During the night a decrease in rapid eye movement (REM) sleep and waking occurs prior to both hot flushes and profuse sweating. Oestrogens alleviate these vasomotor symptoms and improve sleep patterns (Campbell and Whitehead 1977), causing a beneficial domino effect upon minor psychological symptoms.

Oestrogens are readily absorbed through the vaginal skin, causing alleviation of vasomotor symptoms (Dyer *et al.* 1982) and an increase in plasma oestrogen levels. It is therefore essential to use progestogens to prevent the development of endometrial abnormalities.

Women who undergo an earlier menopause are more likely to suffer with ischaemic heart disease (Robinson *et al.* 1959). Replacement oestrogens counteract the adverse changes in plasma lipids which are probably responsible.

REFERENCES

Bungay, G.T., Vessey, M.P. and McPherson, C.K. (1980) Study of symptoms in middle life with special reference to the menopause. *BMJ* ii, 181-3

Campbell, S. and Whitehead, M.I. (1977) 'Oestrogen therapy and the menopausal syndrome' in R. Greenblatt and J.W.W. Studd (Eds) *The Menopause. Clinics in Obstetrics and Gynaecology* 4, pp. 31-7. London: W.B. Saunders

Dyler, G., Townsend, P.T., Jelowitz, J. *et al.* (1982) Dose related changes in vaginal cytology after topical conjugated equine oestrogens. *BMJ* **284**, 789-90

Hunter, M., Battersby, R. and Whitehead, M.I. (1986) Relationships between psychological symptoms, somatic complaints and menopausal status. *Maturitas* **8**, 217-28

Robinson, R.W., Higano, N. and Cohen, W.D. (1959) Increased incidence of coronary heart disease in women castrated prior to the menopause. *Arch Int Med* **104**, 908-13

65 A 43-year-old West African woman complains of very heavy regular periods. She also has dysmenorrhoea and severe premenstrual syndrome (PMS) with suicidal thoughts. Examination reveals a 15-week size fibroid. She is a well-informed patient and for cultural reasons would prefer to retain her uterus if at all possible. The most appropriate management would include the following:

A) Myomectomy. — FALSE
B) Gonadotrophin releasing hormone (GnRH) analogues. — FALSE
C) Counselling followed by total abdominal hysterectomy and bilateral salpingo-oophorectomy and unopposed oestrogen replacement therapy. — TRUE
D) Transcervical endometrial resection. — FALSE
E) Hysterectomy with ovarian conservation. — FALSE

COMMENTS

Although women of African origin very often are reluctant to lose their uterus, this patient would probably accept hysterectomy if counselled appropriately. Hysterectomy alone would, of course, cure her menorrhagia and probably her dysmenorrhoea. It would not cure her premenstrual syndrome which is dependent on ovarian cyclical activity (Backstrom *et al.* 1981). The symptoms of PMS are severe and would justify oophorectomy (Casson *et al.* 1989). It is important to ascertain that the symptoms are present only in the luteal phase of the cycle and that she is not continually depressed. It may be worth testing the potential effect of the oophorectomy on the PMS symptoms by administering GnRH analogue depot for three months.

GnRH would not be the definitive treatment. It would probably stop all of her symptoms but would only reduce the size of the fibroid by about 25%. Additionally, treatment duration would be limited because of the risks of hypoestrogenism, including osteoporosis, cardiovascular disease and menopausal symptoms. Although transcervical endometrial resection would be expected to improve the menorrhagia, there would be no benefit for the pain or the PMS; there are some anecdotal reports of improvement of PMS but these have yet to be confirmed. Total hysterectomy with removal of both ovaries would be most appropriate. The resulting hypoestrogenism can be prevented by giving unopposed oestrogen replacement. In the absence of the uterus (and hence endometrium), progestogen is unnecessary. This is important, as progestogen very often restimulates the PMS symptoms (Magos *et al.* 1986).

REFERENCES

Backstrom, T., Boyle, H. and Baird, D.T. (1981) Persistence of symptoms of premenstrual tension in hysterectomised women. *Br J Obstet Gynaecol* **88**, 530-6

Casson, M.D., Hahn, P.M., Van Vugt, D.A. *et al.* (1989) Lasting response to ovariectomy in severe intractable premenstrual syndrome. *Am J Obstet Gynecol* **162**, 99-105

Magos, A.L., Brewster, E., Singh, R. *et al.* (1986) The effects of norethisterone in postmenopausal women on oestrogen replacement therapy: a model for the premenstrual syndrome. *Br J Obstet Gynaecol* **93**, 1290-6

66 A 35-year-old nulliparous woman presents with a five-year history of primary infertility associated with dysmenorrhoea and pelvic pain. At laparoscopy she is found to have Stage I endometriosis (American Fertility Society Classification). This is the only abnormality detected in the routine investigation of her infertility. The following statements are correct:

A) Medical treatment with danazol or a gonadotrophin releasing-hormone (GnRH) agonist will increase her chances of pregnancy.   FALSE

B) The dysmenorrhoea is likely to resolve with a non-steroidal anti-inflammatory agent.   FALSE

C) *In vitro* fertilisation is less likely to be effective than in a woman of the same age without endometriosis.   TRUE

D) If the disease is left untreated it is unlikely to progress.   FALSE

E) Oestrogen replacement therapy would be contraindicated should she decide to have a hysterectomy and bilateral oophorectomy to treat her pain and dysmenorrhoea.   FALSE

COMMENTS

There is much controversy as to the role mild endometriosis plays in infertility. Endometriosis occurs commonly in fertile women and there is doubt as to whether treatment actually increases the pregnancy rate over those left untreated (Hull *et al.* 1987). It is possible that both the appearance of endometriosis and the infertility are manifestations of the same underlying pathology since the pregnancy rate in those treated remains less than the normal population. Many abnormalities in almost every step of the reproductive process have been demonstrated and it appears that the success rate after *in vitro* fertilisation remains less than in those with no demonstrable disease. Pregnancy was thought to be curative, but it has been demonstrated that the disease will regress spontaneously and it is possible it is these women who become pregnant. However, the reverse has also been documented and in nearly half the women the disease appears to progress (Thomas and Prentice 1992). Dysmenorrhoea is a very common symptom but appears much less successfully treated with the prostaglandin-synthetase inhibitors than primary dysmenorrhoea for reasons unknown. Theoretically oestrogen replacement should be contraindicated particularly in those with severe disease since the endometriosis is oestrogen dependent. There is, however, no good evidence that recurrence is common and so most advocate the use of HRT to prevent postmenopausal side-effects, although it might be advisable to wait a few months before starting treatment. It is possible that the doses of oestrogen in HRT are too low to reactivate disease.

REFERENCES

Hull, M.E., Moghessi, D.F., Magyar, D.F. *et al.* (1987) Comparison of different modalities of endometriosis in infertile women. *Fertil Steril* **47**, 40-4

Thomas, E.J. and Prentice, A. (1992) The aetiology and pathogenesis of endometriosis. *Reprod Med Reviews* **1**, 21-36

67 **A 19-year-old woman presents to her GP with vaginal bleeding and lower abdominal pain two weeks after suction termination of pregnancy (STOP) at ten weeks. The following statements are correct:**

A) Bowel injury secondary to uterine perforation at time of surgery is a likely diagnosis. FALSE

B) Vaginal examination should not be performed before ultrasound scanning to exclude ectopic pregnancy. FALSE

C) Prophylactic antibiotics have not been shown to reduce post-abortion morbidity. FALSE

D) Fifty per cent of patients will develop post-abortion PID if asymptomatic *Chlamydia trachomatis* is isolated from the cervix prior to surgery. TRUE

E) Bacterial vaginosis (anaerobic vaginosis) is present in 10% of asymptomatic patients presenting for TOP. FALSE

COMMENTS

Uterine perforation in itself is not particularly significant unless associated with inadvertent use of instruments (notably the suction evacuation equipment) in the abdominal cavity. Bowel injury may be suspected at the time of the procedure and if unrecognised will present as an acute abdomen over the next 2–4 days.

Ectopic pregnancy co-existing with intrauterine pregnancy is very rare and need not be considered as a likely initial differential diagnosis. Persistence of a positive pregnancy test and umbilical pelvic tenderness ± mass may point to this diagnosis. Vaginal ultrasound scanning may be helpful in assessing retained products of conception following incomplete STOP but is not essential as this diagnosis can usually be made clinically.

Appropriate prophylactic antibiotics have clearly been shown to reduce post-abortion pelvic sepsis. If not used the incidence of moderate to severe post-abortion pelvic sepsis is likely to be around 5-10%.

There is increasing evidence to suggest that mixed anaerobic infection in the vagina is at least as important as *Chlamydia* as a marker for post-abortion pelvic sepsis. Asymptomatic carrier rates in this group of patients is in the region of 20–30%. A lower figure is found at the same gestation in antenatal booking clinics.

The combination of anaerobes plus *Chlamydia* present in the cervix prior to termination of pregnancy is associated with 50% incidence of moderate to severe post-operative pelvic sepsis.

APPROPRIATE READING

Larsson, P.G., Platz-Christensen, J.J., Thejls, H. *et al.* (1992) Incidence of pelvic inflammatory disease after first- trimester legal abortion in women with bacterial vaginosis after treatment with metronidazole: a double-blind, randomized study. *Am J Obstet Gynecol* **166**, 100-3

Larsson, P.G. (1992) Bacterial vaginosis. Diagnosis, treatment and significance in gynaecological practice. *Acta Obstet Gynecol Scand* **71**, 560-1

68 A young woman of 18 years is referred for an urgent opinion because of a three-week history of lower abdominal pain. Her menstrual cycle has been regular, and her LMP two weeks previously. On clinical examination there is lower abdominal tenderness. On bimanual examination cervical excitation pain is elicited, with tenderness in each fornix but no palpable swelling. There is purulent vaginal discharge. For her management:

A) There is adequate evidence to make a confident diagnosis of pelvic inflammatory disease (PID).   FALSE
B) Diagnostic laparoscopy is essential before a diagnosis can be made.   FALSE
C) If the diagnosis is that of PID, the most likely causative agent is *C. trachomatis*.   TRUE
D) Single antibiotic treatment of PID, for example with a cephalosporin, is acceptable, providing there is a rapid clinical response to treatment.   FALSE
E) If the condition was PID and the causative agent was shown to be *Neisseria gonorrhoeae*, the outcome relating to fertility is likely to be better than if the condition had been Chlamydial PID.   TRUE

COMMENTS

The clinical picture given is a common one, and according to Westrom (1988) only 50% of such cases will have PID. Further confirmation should be sought. Valuable symptoms and signs are:

1 Temperature of 38°C or more.

2 Palpable, painful adnexal swelling, if possible confirmed by ultrasound.

3 Intermenstrual bleeding.

4 Raised ESR (greater than 15 mm/hr).

5 Raised WBC (greater than 10 000/mm^3).

6 Positive C. reactive protein test.

7 Positive tests for *N. gonorrhoeae* or *C. trachomatis*.

With one extra diagnostic feature accuracy will rise to 70%, with two extra features to 80% and with three to 96%.

For practical purposes diagnostic laparoscopy is not universally needed, although it is always a useful investigation. It should always be used when the picture is inadequate for a full diagnosis or when other diagnoses are equally possible. It is essential when there is a poor response to treatment after a presumptive diagnosis, and is desirable in older women because of the increased risk of ovarian malignancy.

Sellors *et al.* (1991) have questioned the sensitivity of laparoscopy, which in their series was only 50% accurate. It may be wise to treat some cases with antibiotics even if no disease is shown on laparoscopy.

In Europe 75% of PID cases are initially due to a sexually transmitted agent. *C. trachomatis* is the agent most commonly involved, responsible for up to 50% of all cases (Westrom 1988).

Most cases of PID are polymicrobial in nature, and there is no single antibiotic which provides adequate cover (Soper 1992). Treatment should be with two or even three agents, especially if the results of microbiological tests are not available before prescribing. When mixed infections are due to *C. trachomatis* and other organisms, treatment with agents such as cephalosporins which will not affect *C. trachomatis* may produce partial or complete relief of symptoms (Sweet *et al.* 1983).

Gonococcal PID has always been known to have a better outcome than non-gonococcal PID. Chlamydial PID is more likely to have a poor outcome, perhaps because of the chronicity of the condition (Brunham *et al.* 1988).

REFERENCES

Brunham, R.C., Binns, B. and Guigan, F. (1988) Etiology and outcome of pelvic inflammatory disease. *J Infect Dis* **158**, 510-17

Sellors, J., Mahoney, J., Goldsmith, C. *et al.* (1991) The accuracy of clinical findings and laparoscopy in PID. *Am J Obstet Gynecol* **164**, 113-20

Soper, D.E. (1992) 'Treatment of pelvic inflammatory disease' in G.S. Berger and L.V. Westrom (Eds) *Pelvic Inflammatory Disease*, pp. 87-100. New York: Raven Press

Sweet, R.L., Schecter, J. and Robbie, M.O. (1983) Failure of beta lactor antibiotics to eradicate *C. trachomatis* in the endometrium despite apparent clinical cure of salpingitis. *JAMA* **158**, 2641-5

Westrom, L.V. (1988) 'Long-term consequences of pelvic inflammatory disease' in M.J. Hare (Ed.) *Genital Tract Infection in Women*, pp. 350-67. Edinburgh: Churchill Livingstone

69   The oestrogen in hormone replacement therapy (HRT) in postmenopausal women:

A)	Lowers low-density lipoprotein.	TRUE
B)	Increases the risk of myocardial infarction by approximately 10%.	FALSE
C)	Increases the risk of stroke by more than 15%.	FALSE
D)	Will cause fibroids to enlarge in most women.	FALSE
E)	Causes weight gain.	FALSE

COMMENTS

The oestrogen in HRT, whether delivered orally, transdermally or by implant, has been shown to reduce low-density lipoproteins in postmenopausal women in the majority of published studies. This effect is partly responsible for the observed differences in the incidence of myocardial infarction and stroke between HRT users and non-users. Oestrogen HRT probably reduces the risk of myocardial infarction by approximately 50% and stroke by 20-40%.

Fibroids are common in premenopausal women and regress at the time of the menopause. This is less likely with women taking HRT. There are no published studies of the effects of HRT on fibroid size but anecdotal reports and the experience of hospital menopause clinics with large numbers of patients indicate that fibroids usually remain at the premenopausal size. They seldom enlarge sufficiently to require HRT to be stopped, or hysterectomy.

Numerous controlled studies have shown that oestrogen HRT does not cause greater weight gain than placebo.

APPROPRIATE READING

Bush, T.L., Barrett-Connor, E., Cowan, L.D. *et al.* (1987) Cardiovascular mortality and non-contraceptive use of estrogen in women: results from the Lipid Research Clinics Program Follow-Up Study. *Circulation* **75**, 1102-9

Colditz, G.A. and Stampfer, M.J. (1991) Estrogen replacement therapy and coronary heart disease: a quantitative assessment of the epidemiological evidence. *Prev Med* **20**, 47-63

Colditz, G.A. and Stampfer, M.J. (1992) 'Cardiovascular effects of menopause and estrogen replacement: the epidemiological evidence' in D.P. Swartz (Ed.) *Hormone Replacement Therapy*, pp. 109-37. Baltimore: Williams and Wilkins

Crook, D., Godsland, I.F. and Wynn, V. (1988) 'Ovarian hormones and plasma lipoproteins' in J.W.W. Studd and M.I. Whitehead (Eds) *The Menopause*, pp. 168-80. Oxford: Blackwell Scientific

70 Gonadotrophin releasing hormone (GnRH) agonists:

A) Are derivatives of hypothalamic GnRH with peptide substitution occurring at positions 6 and 12 in amino acid structure.   FALSE
B) Are 20–40 times more potent than native GnRH.   FALSE
C) Will be rapidly deactivated by gastric secretions.   TRUE
D) Will cause maximum fibroid regression by the end of three months' therapy.   TRUE
E) Induce suppression of gonadotrophin levels within seven days of treatment.   TRUE

COMMENTS

The peptide substitutions are at positions 6 and 10 and these substitutions mean that the analogues are from 40 to 200 times more potent than native GnRH because of an increased binding affinity to pituitary GnRH receptors and increased peptidase degradation (McLaghlan *et al.* 1986). The peptides are rapidly deactivated by gastric secretions and are most commonly administered by nasal sprays, slow-release intramuscular preparations of microspheres or implants given at monthly intervals.

Treatment of fibroids with GnRH analogues leads to approximately 50% reduction of initial volume. Maximum regression occurs by the end of three months of therapy which, if continued, leads to no further significant shrinkage (William and Shaw 1990).

Initial exposure to GnRH analogues induces stimulation of serum gonadotrophins accompanied by increased concentration of steroids. However, with continued administration, in 5–6 days gonadotrophin levels return to pretreatment levels and become further suppressed, often to below follicular phase values (Fraser 1988).

REFERENCES

Fraser, H. (1988) LHRH analogues: their clinical physiology and delivery systems. *Baillière's Clin Obstet Gynaecol* 2, 639-58

McLaghlan, R., Healy, D. and Burger, H. (1986) Clinical aspects of LHRH analogues in gynaecology: a review. *Br J Obstet Gynaecol* **99**, 431-54

William, I. and Shaw, I. (1990) Effect of naferelin on uterine fibroids measured by ultrasound and NMR. *Eur J Obstet Gynecol* **34**, 111-17

71 Psychological symptoms associated with the climacteric:

A) Include memory loss and inability to concentrate.   TRUE

B) That improve with hormone replacement therapy are always accompanied by hot flushes.   FALSE

C) Are commoner in women who do not attend menopause clinics.   FALSE

D) May be worsened with oestrogen hormone replacement therapy (HRT).   FALSE

E) May account for the increased risk of suicide reported in HRT users. TRUE

COMMENTS

Psychological disturbances at the time of the climacteric include poor memory, inability to concentrate, loss of confidence, irritability and emotional lability. HRT will often improve these symptoms and sometimes this results from an improvement in flushes. However, there are reports of these symptoms improving with HRT in women who do not have hot flushes.

Psychological symptoms are commoner in women who attend menopause clinics, as they are in outpatient attenders in general. The UK MRC study reported an increased incidence of suicide in HRT users.

There are no reports of HRT worsening climacteric psychological symptoms. The common side-effects of oestrogens are breast tenderness and leg cramps. Progestogens may cause side-effects similar to the symptoms of the premenstrual syndrome.

APPROPRIATE READING

Campbell, S. and Whitehead, M.I. (1977) Oestrogen therapy and the menopausal syndrome. *Clin Obstet Gynaecol* **4** , 31-47

Gath, D. and Iles, S. (1990) 'Psychological effects of the menopause' in J.O. Drife and J.W.W. Studd (Eds) *HRT and Osteoporosis*, pp. 34-45. London: Springer-Verlag

Hunt, K., Vessey, M. and McPherson, K. (1990) Mortality in a cohort of long-term users of hormone replacement therapy: an updated analysis. *Br J Obstet Gynaecol* **97**, 1080-6

Marsh, M.S. and M.I. Whitehead (1992) Management of the menopause. *Br Med Bull* **48**, 426-7

72 Menorrhagia can be diagnosed accurately:

A) By measuring the endometrial thickness at ultrasound.   FALSE
B) From a detailed history from the patient regarding quantity of sanitary protection.   FALSE
C) When there is a history of flooding and clots.   FALSE
D) By hysteroscopy and endometrial sampling.   FALSE
E) From a full blood count.   FALSE

COMMENTS

The diagnosis of menorrhagia is made when the loss per cycle exceeds the 90th centile for the population, that is, greater than 80 ml (Hallberg *et al.* 1966). The simpler methods of diagnosing menorrhagia are inadequate. It is probably true to say that a significant proportion of women having hysterectomy for heavy periods have their operation when their loss is normal (Coulter *et al.* 1988). The patient's impression of her loss, the quantity of sanitary protection used, the duration of bleeding, the presence of clots and flooding and the use of the simpler menstrual charts are of no value in quantifying an individual patient's loss.

Attempts to weigh tampons and pads or to measure uterine size or endometrial thickness have proved equally valueless (Chimbira *et al.* 1980; Fraser *et al.* 1984).

Hysteroscopy and endometrial sampling may be important in such patients but of course this is to detect associated pathology and does not assist in the diagnosis of menorrhagia. Haemoglobin estimation is important in these patients, but patients frequently have menorrhagia but maintain their haemoglobin. A normal haemoglobin does not exclude menorrhagia. One method which has become the 'gold standard' is the alkaline haematein technique; although this is cumbersome and time consuming it is precise (Hallberg *et al.* 1966). A newer, much simpler technique using the pictorial blood-loss assessment chart correlates well with the alkaline haematein method and is far simpler and thus most appropriate for clinical use (Higham *et al.* 1990).

REFERENCES

Chimbira, T.H., Anderson, A.B. and Turnbull, A.C. (1980) Relationship between measured menstrual blood loss and patients' subjective assessment of loss, duration of bleeding, number of sanitary towels, uterine weight, and endometrial surface area. *Br J Obstet Gynaecol* **87**, 603-9

Coulter, A., McPherson, K. and Vessey, M. (1988) Do British women undergo too many hysterectomies? *Soc Sci Med* **17**, 987-94

Fraser, I., McCarron, G. and Markham, R. (1984) A preliminary study of factors influencing the perception of menstrual blood loss volume. *Am J Obstet Gynecol* **149**, 788-93

Hallberg, A., Hogdahl, A., Nilsson, L. *et al.* (1966) Menstrual blood loss; a population study. *Acta Obstet Gynecol Scand* **45**, 320-51

Higham, J., O'Brien, P.M.S. and Shaw, R.W. (1990) Assessment of menstrual blood loss using a pictorial chart. *Br J Obstet Gynaecol* **97**, 734-9

73 **A 24-year-old woman presents with a 3 cm ovarian cyst which is asymptomatic. At laparoscopy it is found to be an endometrioma. No other coloured lesions are present in the peritoneal cavity. Which of the following statements are correct?**

A) This may be treated successfully with a gonadotrophin releasing hormone (GnRH) agonist.   FALSE
B) The absence of coloured lesions indicates the absence of other endometriotic tissue.   FALSE
C) This patient is likely to have impaired fertility.   TRUE
D) Treatment requires laparotomy for adequate cyst removal.   FALSE
E) The ovary containing the endometrioma should be removed.   FALSE

COMMENTS

These cysts may be treated at the time of laparoscopy. The contents are extremely irritant and must be carefully aspirated and peritoneal lavage performed. The cyst should then be excised. There is no need to remove the ovary (Sutton 1991). The capsule contains endometriotic tissue which must be removed using dissection and diathermy or vaporised using laser. Laparotomy is necessary if the surgeon is unexperienced in laparoscopic surgery as medical treatment is unlikely to have any effect on this type of lesion. There is now evidence that endometriosis may be white, colourless or even invisible since apparently normal endometrium can contain endometriotic tissue (Donnez *et al.* 1990). It is possible that these are early lesions which then progress through the typical red, flame-like lesions to the inactive, black powder spots. Endometriosis associated with anatomical distortion is likely to be associated with infertility although the situation with mild disease is unclear.

REFERENCES

Donnez, J., Nisolle, M., Casanas-Roux, F. *et al.* (1990) 'Endometriosis: pathogenesis and pathophysiology' in R.W. Shaw (Ed.) *Endometriosis*, pp. 11-30. Carnforth: Parthenon Publishing

Sutton, C. (1991) 'The treatment of endometriosis' in J. Studd (Ed.) *Progress in Obstetrics and Gynaecology*, **8**, pp. 251-72. Edinburgh: Churchill Livingstone

FURTHER READING

Schweppe, K.W. (1990) 'Current medical therapies for endometriosis: a review' in R.W. Shaw (Ed.) *Endometriosis*, pp. 67-84. Carnforth: Parthenon Publishing

74   Which of the following statements with regard to the combined pill (COC) are correct?

A) If a woman has had a splenectomy for any reason and the platelet count is above $500 \times 10^9/l$, this contraindicates the combined pill.   TRUE

B) The COC pill increases the incidence of candidiasis.   FALSE

C) Women with severe inflammatory bowel disease (ulcerative colitis or Crohn's) should avoid oestrogen containing pills.   TRUE

D) There is no need to investigate or treat secondary amenorrhoea lasting six months if it followed discontinuation of the COC (sometimes termed 'post-pill' amenorrhoea).   FALSE

E) It is generally preferable for women taking the COC to take a six months' break in use after about ten years.   FALSE

COMMENTS

Splenectomy is often overlooked as a potential risk factor for thrombosis. It may have been indicated through trauma or as part of treatment for conditions such as thalassaemia major or spherocytosis. In most cases any post-splenectomy thrombocytosis is transient and the platelet count then remains within the normal range, 150-400×10^9 per litre. The count should be monitored and if it rises above 500×10^9 this increases the risk especially of arterial thrombosis – which might be exacerbated by the small but well-established prothrombotic changes caused by oestrogen (Guillebaud 1989).

The title of a study in the *British Journal of Obstetrics and Gynaecology* involving over 1300 women says it all: 'The pill does not cause thrush' (Davidson and Oates 1985). Modern low-oestrogen pills do not increase the rate of this common condition above background.

There are numerous reports of thromboembolism during severe (hospitalised) exacerbations of ulcerative colitis and Crohn's diseases. Should these occur the COC pill should be discontinued during attacks, and any woman who is prone to repeated bad attacks should avoid oestrogen altogether. During prolonged remissions, however, the method is only relatively contraindicated since there is no problem with absorption of the artificial hormones. This has been found to be entirely within normal limits in both conditions, even in women with ileostomies (Grimmer *et al.* 1986).

Combined pill takers who develop Crohn's disease for the first time should be given a trial without the method since the COC has been associated (probably causally) with the development of non-granulomatous Crohn's (Rhodes *et al.* 1984).

The term 'post-pill' amenorrhoea should be abolished, since most authorities now believe any association with the COC is casual not causal. Amenorrhoea of more than six months' duration occurs in about 2% of the population. If a woman is predisposed but instead takes the COC for many years, any episodes that would otherwise have been recognised will be masked by the regular withdrawal bleeds induced by her contraceptive. In such a woman, the pill is easily blamed for her 'after pill' secondary amenorrhoea when it could, after all, only be revealed 'after pill' (Jacobs 1987).

Moreover, studies show that the probability of this amenorrhoea is not associated with formulation, nor with duration of use. Professor Jacobs and co-workers at the UCH School of Medicine in London have shown that the distribution of diagnoses was the same in cases of secondary amenorrhoea post-pill as in non-post-pill cases; and in the two groups the types of treatment needed, and the excellent outcome in terms of cumulative conception rates were all the same (Hull *et al.* 1981). Thus there is no specific pill-induced syndrome causing secondary amenorrhoea, and after six months without a period all cases of secondary amenorrhoea should be referred for investigation and appropriate treatment.

Another unfortunate result of accepting post-pill amenorrhoea as a real condition is that it deters doctors from prescribing COCs to women for whom they otherwise might be suitable or even preferable. A past history of secondary amenorrhoea, now resolved, is a good example. But in many cases of oligo-amenorrhoea the COC pill can be positively beneficial: when there is hypo-oestrogenism; or in the polycystic ovary syndrome where it can control androgenic symptoms (Jacobs 1987) and so improve the potentially atherogenic lipid profile while also protecting the endometrium from overstimulation and the risk of neoplasia.

For most sexually active women, on a careful assessment of the balance of risks and benefits, it would be preferable not to take short breaks after any arbitrary time. If the break itself is prolonged, there may be a benefit to adverse effects such as breast cancer risk in the young, but the enhancement by longer durations of use to established beneficial effects of the COC (e.g. on ovarian cancer risk) will also be lost. Six-month breaks are too short to influence total accumulated duration of use significantly, but quite long enough to lead to many unwanted pregnancies.

Data suggest that the regular pill-free 'break' may be beneficial: HDL-cholesterol suppression which was at its peak on the 21st day of pill-taking was back in the normal range at the end of the pill-free interval (Demacker et al. 1982). Guillebaud (1989) hypothesises that the 130 'breaks' which a woman who has been on the pill for ten years has already had may well be sufficient to prevent excessive metabolic changes. They also seem to be enough to ensure excellent reversibility in ex-users.

The above does not imply that women should be forced to continue taking the pill against their own inclinations. The usual reason for requesting a break is because their friends have suggested it. However if, after discussion on the above lines, they still feel the need for a break irrespective of peer group pressure, then an effective alternative should of course be arranged.

REFERENCES

Davidson, F. and Oates, J.K. (1985) The pill does not cause 'thrush'. *Br J Obstet Gynaecol* **92**, 1265-6

Demacker, P.N., Schade, R.W., Stalenhoef, A.F. *et al.* (1982) Influence of contraceptive pill and menstrual cycle on serum lipids and high-density lipoprotein cholesterol concentrations. *BMJ* **284**, 1213-15

Grimmer, S.F., Back, D.J., Orme, M.L. *et al.* (1986) The bioavailability of ethinyloestradiol and levonorgestrel in patients with an ileostomy. *Contraception* **33**, 51-9

Guillebaud, J. (1989) 'Practical prescribing of combined oral contraceptive pill' in M. Filshie and J. Guillebaud (Eds) *Contraception: Science and Practice*, pp. 69-93. London: Butterworth Heinemann

Hull, M.J., Bromham, D.R., Savage, P.E. *et al.* (1981) Normal fertility in women with post-pill amenorrhoea. *Lancet* **i**, 1229-32

Jacobs, H.S. (1987) The care of patients with past and present amenorrhoea. *Br J Fam Plann* **12** (suppl), 2-5

Rhodes, J.M., Cockel, R., Allan, R.N. *et al.* (1984) Colonic Crohn's disease and use of oral contraception. *BMJ* **288**, 595-6

Talbot, R.W., Heppell, J., Dozois, R.R. *et al.* (1986) Vascular complications of inflammatory bowel disease. *Mayo Clin Proc* **61**, 140-5

75 It has been suggested that a male factor is at least partly responsible for 30–50% of infertility in couples presenting to a specialist clinic. Important amongst the causes of male factor infertility are disorders of spermatogenesis. Which of the following may be associated with an irreversible impairment of spermatogenesis?

A) Excessive intake of alcohol.	TRUE
B) Anabolic steroids.	FALSE
C) Mumps orchitis.	TRUE
D) Sulphasalazine prescribed for the treatment of ulcerative colitis.	FALSE
E) Klinefelter (XYY) syndrome.	TRUE

COMMENTS

It has been estimated that approximately one in seven couples in the UK of reproductive age who desire pregnancy are unable to conceive within 12 months. Initial consultation should include history and physical examination, assessment of testicular descent, size and consistency, noting varicoceles and other abnormalities, e.g. hypospadias.

A semen sample should be analysed ideally within one hour of ejaculation. WHO classification of standard values sperm density $>20 \times 10^6$/ml, motility $>50\%$, normal morphology $>60\%$. White blood cells should be $<1 \times 10^6$. Three semen analyses should be undertaken within 90 days. Further assessment may include: sperm penetration assay or zona-free hamster egg assay. Human oocyte fertilisation rate, the 24-hour sperm survival test following swim-up or sperm wash and computerised analysis of sperm movement patterns. Recent experience with IVF has suggested that some men with apparently normal semen parameters may be infertile.

Causes of male factor infertility include disorders of spermatogenesis which may be pretesticular or testicular. A history of cryptorchidism is significant as in addition to being deleterious to spermatogenesis there may be associated epididymal abnormalities. Other urinary tract congenital anomalies and a history of previous surgery should be sought, particularly hernia or hydrocele repair. Mumps orchitis/acute testicular injury/inflammation may result in destruction or sclerosis of seminiferous tubules. Recurrent urinary tract infection, prostatitis or haemospermia require investigation and treatment as bacteria may adversely affect sperm function.

Drug use/abuse may temporarily depress spermatogenesis, particularly those prescribed for urinary tract infection or ulcerative colitis. Excessive use of alcohol suppresses spermatogenesis by a direct testicular effect and has a secondary effect by virtue of liver dysfunction. Other drugs of addiction including smoking may affect sperm function directly. Anabolic steroids are known to suppress testicular function and consequently impair spermatogenesis. Semen analysis should be repeated three months after discontinuation of drugs or recent acute or prolonged illness.

Effective treatment may be divided into the following categories – surgery aimed at specific physical defects, e.g. varicoceles, microsurgical techniques for obstructive azoospermia. Congenital absence of the vas or scarring of the epididymides are not amenable to surgical correction. However, initial experience with microepididymal sperm aspiration (MESA) combined with zygote intra-fallopian transfer/IVF is promising. Endocrine-related infertility, e.g. hyperprolactinaemia and hypogonadotrophic hypogonadism respond to specific treatment.

Artificial insemination is generally disappointing except for male impotence and severe hypospadias. Variable fertilisation and pregnancy rates are recorded for IVF/ET. Recent innovations, e.g. microinjection sperm transfer techniques, the use of additives such as pentoxyfylline, are promising but need to be adequately assessed.

APPROPRIATE READING

Aitken, R.J., Sutton, M., Warner, P. *et al.* (1985) Relationship between the movement characteristics of human spermatozoa and their ability to penetrate cervical mucus and zona-free hamster eggs. *J Reprod Fertil* **73**, 441-9

Jequier, A. (1986) 'Infertility in the male' in *Current Reviews in Obstetrics and Gynaecology*. Edinburgh: Churchill Livingstone

World Health Organisation (1987) *WHO Laboratory Manual for the Examination of Human Semen and Semen-cervical Mucus Interaction*. Cambridge: Cambridge University Press

76 **A patient has had four first-trimester abortions. Which of the following investigations might be helpful?**

A) Maternal and paternal HLA typing.	FALSE
B) Maternal and paternal chromosome analysis.	TRUE
C) Hysteroscopy.	TRUE
D) Anti-nuclear factor.	TRUE
E) High vaginal swab.	FALSE

COMMENTS

Initial enthusiasm for parental HLA studies in recurrent abortion (RM) (evidence for increased sharing being aetiologically significant) has failed to reach statistical levels.

Two per cent of couples will reveal a chromosomal abnormality of aetiological significance.

Hysteroscopy should add to the diagnosis of congenital uterine abnormalities causing RM.

Anti-nuclear factor will screen for antiphospholipid antibodies. There is no proof as yet of bacterial vaginosis causing recurrent first-trimester abortion.

SUGGESTED READING

Johnson, P.M. and Ramsden, G.H. (1988) Recurrent miscarriage. *Clin Immunol Allergy*, October, pp. 607-24

77 **Transvaginal sonography has increased the accuracy of ultrasound diagnosis in gynaecology. Which of the following statements are correct?**

A) The demonstration of a gestational sac in the adnexal region of the uterus enables a definite diagnosis of tubal pregnancy to be made.   FALSE

B) An early intrauterine pregnancy should be seen when a serum beta HCG level is 700 iu/l.   TRUE

C) A vaginal scan is contraindicated in patients with acute PID.   FALSE

D) An ultrasound frequency of 7.5 kHz is optimal for transvaginal scanning.   FALSE

E) The average follicular growth rate is 1 mm/day between day 10 of the menstrual cycle and ovulation.   FALSE

COMMENTS

Transvaginal sonography enables the detection of an intact ectopic pregnancy in more than 70% of patients. A definite diagnosis can be made when the ectopic sac contains an embryo or yolk sac. The differentiation between an empty sac and non-specific adnexal pathology including corpus luteum cysts is sometimes difficult and may lead to a false positive diagnosis.

In a study of 22 healthy volunteers who were scanned every 2–4 days after the first positive pregnancy test until a living fetus was observed, a gestational sac 1–3 mm in diameter was detected at a mean of 31.2 days' gestation (range 30–33 days) and at a mean HCG level of 730 iu/l (range 467–935 iu/l).

Pressure is not necessary to perform a vaginal scan, therefore the procedure is not contraindicated in cases of PID.

The optimal frequency of vaginal ultrasound is 5–10 MHz. The mean daily growth rate of the follicle is constant at around 2 mm per day reaching an average size of 20 mm shortly before ovulation.

APPROPRIATE READING

Cacciatore, B., Marrs, P.R., Kletzy, O.A. et al. (1990) Normal early pregnancy: serum HCG levels and vaginal ultrasonography findings. *Br J Obstet Gynaecol* **97**, 899-903

Varygas, J.M., Titinen, A., Stenman, U-H. et al. (1982) Correlation of ultrasonic measurement of ovarian follicle size and serum estradiol levels in ovulatory patients following clomiphene citrate for *in vitro* fertilization. *Am J Obstet Gynecol* **144**, 569-73

78 Which of the following statements about chemotherapy for ovarian carcinoma are correct?

A) In the treatment of advanced ovarian cancer with chemotherapy the dose intensity does not correlate with objective response or with median survival.   FALSE

B) Intraperitoneal administration of cisplatin produces a 30% complete response rate in women with persistent disease after initial treatment of ovarian carcinoma with intravenous cisplatin.   TRUE

C) Taxol is a promising new cytotoxic agent which acts by decreasing levels of intracellular glutathione (GSH).   FALSE

D) Sulphydryl compounds such as WR-2721 protect against the ototoxicity, nephrotoxicity and neuropathy associated with cisplatin therapy.   TRUE

E) The interferons have not demonstrated activity via intravenous or intraperitoneal routes in the management of ovarian carcinoma.   FALSE

COMMENTS

In a review of 33 trials of chemotherapy in advanced ovarian carcinoma, Levin and Hryniuk (1987) found that the dose intensity correlated with both objective response and median survival. Combination chemotherapy was more effective than single agent regimes. Of the single agents, cisplatin is the most active with a high-dose intensity correlation.

Investigators using the intraperitoneal route have shown up to 30% complete responses in women who have had persistent disease following intravenous cisplatin treatment for ovarian carcinoma (Markman *et al.* 1989). This is only evident in women with less than 0.5 cm disease.

Taxol is extracted from the bark of the Pacific yew; it is a promising cytotoxic agent which has been shown to have activity in patients with refractory ovarian carcinoma. Its mode of action is by polymerising tubulin; it is therefore an antimicrotubule agent (McGuire *et al.* 1989).

Certain agents are known to have ameliorating effects against chemotherapy related toxicity. WR-2721 is a sulphydryl which is concentrated in normal tissues and excluded from most neoplastic cells. It acts by protecting against cell damage caused by oxygen free radicals. It reduces the ototoxicity, nephrotoxicity and neuropathy caused by cisplatin and the myelosuppression caused by alkylating agents (Glover *et al.* 1986).

Biological response modifiers have also been studied in the management of ovarian carcinoma. As yet no biological agent has an established, well-defined role but the interferons have shown some activity via both intravenous and intraperitoneal routes in small trials (Markman 1987; McGuire and Rowinsky 1991).

REFERENCES

Glover, D., Glick, J.H., Weiler, C. *et al.* (1986) WR-2721 protects against the hematologic toxicity of cyclophosphamide: a controlled phase 11 trial. *J Clin Oncol* **4**, 584-8

Levin, L. and Hryniuk, W.M. (1987) Dose intensity analysis of chemotherapy regimens in ovarian carcinoma. *J Clin Oncol* **5**, 756-67

Markman, M. (1987) Intracavitary administration of biological agents. *J Biol Response Mod* **6**, 404

Markman, M., Hakes, T., Reichman, B. *et al.* (1989) Intraperitoneal therapy in the management of ovarian carcinoma. *Yale J Biol Med* **62**, 393-403

McGuire, W.P., Rowinsky, E.K., Rosenshein, N.B. *et al.* (1989) Taxol: a unique antineoplastic agent with significant activity in advanced ovarian epithelial neoplasms. *Ann Intern Med* **111**, 273-9

McGuire, W.P. and Rowinsky, E.K. (1991) Old drugs revisited, new drugs and experimental approaches in ovarian cancer therapy. *Semin Oncol* **18**, 255-69

79 Regarding Depo-Provera® (DMPA), which of the following statements are correct about this injectable?

A) It is absolutely contraindicated by a past history of thromboembolism or a 'focal' migraine.   FALSE

B) It is a good choice for the contraceptive needs of a woman before, during and immediately after major surgery or surgery to the leg.   TRUE

C) If a user of Depo-Provera® develops amenorrhoea for more than one year the method should be discontinued because of hypo-oestrogenism and the risk of developing osteoporosis.   FALSE

D) The latest WHO research shows no association in the generality of Depo-Provera® users between its use and the development of primary cancers of the breast, cervix, ovary or liver. TRUE

E) During rifampicin therapy there is no need to increase the dose of each injection but the injection interval should be reduced from 12 weeks to normally every eight weeks.   TRUE

COMMENTS

There is no sound evidence for the statement in the Data Sheet that, 'Depo-Provera® is contraindicated in thrombophlebitis or a history of pulmonary embolism.' Laboratory research has failed to show any significant pro-thrombotic effects of medroxyprogesterone acetate (Whigham *et al.* 1979); no epidemiological risk of thromboembolism has been shown; and the anecdotes of women using this injectable who have suffered thrombotic events are probably explained by predisposition (leading perhaps to them having discontinued oestrogen-containing pills before transferring to the injectable). The *British National Formulary* (1994) mentions severe arterial disease but rightly omits past thromboembolism as (absolute) contraindications. DMPA is, however, *relatively* contraindicated by past thrombosis and should therefore be used advisedly, with full counselling, in view of the possibility that any woman with a past thrombosis may suffer a recurrence.

In *focal* migraine there is transient cerebral ischaemia. The concern, as reported by Bickerstaff (1975), is that the established if small pro-thrombotic effects of oestrogen, even in the modern pills, might be capable of turning a transient ischaemia into a permanent ischaemia (i.e. a stroke) (Guillebaud 1989). This concern about an excess risk due to the contraceptive is eliminated by use of any oestrogen-free method, such as DMPA or the progestogen-only pill (POP); though the woman may continue to get focal migraines.

It is agreed by most authorities that oestrogen should be avoided for four weeks prior to elective major surgery or any surgery to the legs or associated with significant immobilisation, and not recommended until at least two weeks after full mobilisation (Guillebaud 1985). DMPA is at least as effective as the COC pill – thus preventing conception while on the waiting list; moreover, the COC pill can be recommended as convenient without waiting for the full 12 weeks after the last injection to have elapsed.

A cross-sectional comparative study by Cundy *et al.* (1991) showed that DMPA users with amenorrhoea had a slight (about 7%) reduction of lumbar bone density as compared with premenopausal controls. This study has been much criticised and requires prospective confirmation. Pending better data, the recommendation of the British National Association of Family Planning Doctors (NAFPD) (1993) is that after five years of amenorrhoea it is reasonable to arrange for a plasma oestradiol. If the result is more than 100 pmol/l no action need be taken. If it is below this figure a new method may be offered, or in a symptom-free woman at her request the DMPA may be continued, with monitoring. If a bone scan is available and shows suboptimal bone density there can be consideration of 'add back' oestrogen (Premarin® 0.625 mg daily or equivalent), or of oestrogen replacement therapy alone subsequent to the DMPA.

Reassuring findings with regard to human (as opposed to beagle bitch) breast cancer were reported in 1991 (WHO Collaborative Study of Neoplasia and Steroid Contraceptives). The relative risk of DMPA if ever injected was 1.21 (CI 0.96, 1.52). The risk appeared to be increased within the first four years of initial exposure in women under 35 years, but without any duration-of-use effect. This could well have been caused by surveillance bias in DMPA users. There was no increased risk in the other three types of cancer in the question and there was a five-fold reduction in the risk of carcinoma of the endometrium (RR=0.21) (Kaunitz 1992).

Rifampicin is a very powerful inducer of liver enzymes, hence lowering the blood level and area under the curve of both oestrogens and progestogens (Orme and Back 1991). Since the blood profile of DMPA shows high values in the first four weeks, declining thereafter, simply increasing the dose of the initial injection would have a greater effect on the peak blood level than on the duration that the dose was above the threshold to prevent conception. It is therefore now recommended that the injection interval be shortened, as above.

REFERENCES

Bickerstaff, E.R. (1975) *Neurological Complications of Oral Contraceptives*, pp. 16-39; 81-6. Oxford: Oxford University Press

British National Formulary (1992) 27, Section 7.3.2, pp. 305-6. London: British Medical Association/Royal Pharmaceutical Society of Great Britain

Cundy, T., Evans, M., Roberts, H. *et al.* (1991) Bone density in women receiving depot medroxyprogesterone acetate for contraception. *BMJ* **383**, 13-16

Guillebaud, J. (1985) Surgery and the pill. *BMJ* **291**, 498-9

Guillebaud, J. (1989) 'Practical prescribing of the combined oral contraceptive pill' in M. Filshie and J. Guillebaud (Eds) *Contraception: Science and Practice*, pp. 83-5. London: Butterworth Heinemann

Kaunitz, A.M. (1992) Injectable contraception: the USA perspective. *IPPF Med Bull* **26**: 6, 1-3

National Association of Family Planning Doctors (1993) Report of clinical scientific and advisory committee. *Br J Fam Plann* **18**, 134

Orme, M. and Back, D.J. (1991) Oral contraceptive steroids – pharmacological issues of interest to the prescribing physician. *Adv Contr* **7**, 325-31

Whigham, K.A., Howie, P.W., Mack, A. *et al.* (1979) The effect of an injectable contraceptive on blood coagulation and fibrinolysis. *Br J Obstet Gynaecol* **86**, 122-6

WHO Collaborative Study of Neoplasia and Steroid Contraceptives (1991) Breast cancer and depot-medroxyprogesterone acetate: a multinational study. *Lancet* **338**, 833-8

80 A woman of 61 who is ten years postmenopause attends the outpatient clinic complaining of hot flushes and vaginal dryness. Recent dual X-ray absorptometry bone density measurements showed that she has bone density below the age-matched 5th percentile for both the hip and the spine. She is otherwise fit and well. Which of the following statements are correct?

A) Oestrogen HRT will not significantly affect bone density in women over 60 years of age.   FALSE

B) Dietary calcium supplementation is indicated.   FALSE

C) Clonidine may control the hot flushes and preserve bone density.   FALSE

D) Intermittent oral etidronate will reduce the risk of future fracture.   TRUE

E) Progestogen alone may control hot flushes, but will have no effect on bone density.   FALSE

COMMENTS

Oestrogen HRT in adequate dosage will maintain bone density in the majority of postmenopausal women regardless of their age or bone density. Calcium supplements may be of benefit in women who consume less than 500 mg of calcium per day but this is unusual in women consuming a healthy Western diet. Examples of the calcium content of foods include: 235 mg (1/3 pint) skimmed milk; 250 mg (5 oz) yoghourt and 207 mg (10 oz) cheddar cheese.

Clonidine will control hot flushes in some women by acting to stabilise the peripheral vasculature; it has no known or theoretical action on bone density. Etidronate given for two weeks out of every 13 will preserve bone density and has been shown to reduce fracture risk in osteoporotic women. Progestogens alone will reduce cortical bone loss but it is uncertain whether they preserve trabecular bone. The lack of data concerning effects on bone density, their adverse effects on the lipoprotein profile (e.g. lowering high-density lipoprotein) and PMS-type side-effects means that progestogens alone are unsuitable as a long-term alternative to oestrogen HRT.

APPROPRIATE READING

Gallagher, J.C., Kable, W.T. and Goldar, D. (1991) Effect of progestin therapy on cortical and trabecular bone: comparison with estrogen. *Am J Med* **90**, 171-8

Marsh, M.S. and Whitehead, M.I. (1992) Management of the menopause. *Br Med Bull* **48**, 426-57

Stevenson, J.C. and Marsh, M.S. (1992) *An Atlas of Osteoporosis*, p. 104. Carnforth: Partheron Publishing

Storm, T., Thamsborg, G., Steiniche, T. *et al.* (1990) Effect of intermittent cyclical etidronate therapy on bone mass and fracture rate in women with postmenopausal osteoporosis. *N Engl J Med* **322**, 1265-71

Watts, N.B., Harris, S.T., Genant, H.K. *et al.* (1990) Intermittent cyclical etidronate treatment of postmenopausal osteoporosis. *N Engl J Med* **323**, 73-9

81 **Which of the following regimens are known to be effective in preventing pregnancy if given post-coitally?**

A) Two tablets of Ovran® 50 taken twice if separated by twelve hours.	TRUE
B) Twenty-five tablets of Microval® taken twice separated by twelve hours.	TRUE
C) 200 mg danazol taken twice separated by twelve hours.	FALSE
D) 50 mg clomiphene taken twice separated by twelve hours.	FALSE
E) 10 mg GnRH antagonist given once IM.	FALSE

COMMENTS

The standard regimen for post-coital contraception (PCC) licensed in the UK since 1984 is a combination of 100 μg ethinyl-oestradiol and 1 mg dl norgestrel (COC). While the combination is specifically marketed as a PCC (Schering PC4®) it is much cheaper to prescribe 4 × 50 μg combined oral contraceptive pills and provided the pills are properly packaged and instructions for use appended this is perfectly acceptable practice. Because COC is associated with a high incidence of side-effects other agents have been tried. Norethisterone 0.75 mg given twice 12 hours apart has been shown to have a similar failure rate as COC (Ho 1992). It is marketed in many Asian and some East European countries as Postinor but is not available as a proprietary preparation in the UK. Microval® is a gestogen-only pill consisting of 30 μg levonorgestrel; 25 tablets are equivalent to 0.75 mg.

There is some doubt as to whether danazol is an effective post-coital agent. Two UK studies (Rowlands et al. 1986; Webb et al. 1992) showed quite high failure rates while an Italian study of high doses of danazol (Zuliani et al. 1990) reported failure rates which were as good as, or better than, COC. 200 mg twice has not been tested but is probably not enough. Clomiphene is an anti-oestrogen which is used for inducing ovulation. Oestrogen is probably not essential for implantation in the human although there is some evidence to suggest that clomiphene may prevent pregnancy in the monkey (Ravindranth and Mougdal 1987).

There is a lot of interest in GnRH antagonists as contraceptives. The corpus luteum is dependent on LH and in theory a luteolytic agent which inhibits LH binding should be an effective post-coital agent. While a single dose of the GnRH antagonist does cause a drop in progesterone secretion from the corpus luteum (CL), the CL can be rescued by the administration of HCG (Bouchard 1991) so that the window of opportunity for the antagonist effectively to inhibit implantation is too small to be clinically promising.

REFERENCES

Bouchard, P. (1991) 'Potential clinical applications of antagonists' in C.M. Howles (Ed.) *Gonadotrophins, Gonadotrophin-releasing Hormone Analogues and Growth Factors in Fertility: Future Perspectives*. (Proc. meeting in Harrogate, UK, 29-30 April 1991. Serono Seminars.) Oxford: Alden Press

Ho, P.C. (1992) Asian experience with post coital contraception. *Adv Contraception* **8**, 216

Ravindranth, N. and Mougdal, N.R. (1987) Use of tamoxifen, an anti-oestrogen, in establishing a need for oestrogen in early pregnancy in the Bonnet monkey (*Macaca radiata*). *J Reprod Fertil* **81**, 327-36

Rowlands, S., Kubba, A.A., Guillebaud, J. *et al.* (1986) A possible mechanism of action of danazol and an ethinyloestradiol/norgestrel combination used as post-coital contraceptive agents. *Contraception* **33**, 539-45

Webb, A.M.C., Russel, J. and Elstein, M. (1992) Comparison of the Yuzpe regimen, danazol and mifepristone in oral post-coital contraception. *BMJ* **305**, 927-31

Zuliani, G., Coluombo, U.F. and Molla, R. (1990) Hormonal post-coital contraception with an ethinylestradiol-norgestrel combination and two danazol regimens. *Eur J Obstet Gynecol Reprod Biol* **37**, 253-60

82 Failure of fertilisation of human oocyte in an IVF programme may:

A) Occur only when the capacitation process is complete.   FALSE
B) Be demonstrated by the presence of glycoproteins termed 'decapacitation factors'.   TRUE
C) Occur more commonly with mature oocytes than with immature/atretic oocytes.   FALSE
D) Be due to failure of induction of the sperm acrosome reaction.   TRUE
E) Be an indication for micromanipulation of oocytes (e.g. sub-zonal insemination) in subsequent attempts at IVF.   TRUE

COMMENTS

Capacitation is the process by which epididymal sperm, after ejaculation, undergoes further modification. This can occur either in the female genital tract or *in vitro*. In the human female genital tract the process involves the elimination of the constituents of seminal plasma from the surface of the sperm as it traverses the cervical canal and the uterine lumen (Lambert *et al.* 1985; Plachot and Mandelbaum 1990). Capacitation can also occur *in vitro*, without the help of the female genital tract, and this can occur in as short a period as one hour (Plachot *et al.* 1985).

The process of capacitation *in vitro* is induced by removing sperm from seminal plasma, and by washing and incubating these sperm in culture medium. During this process, certain cell surface components, namely glycoproteins, are altered or modified. In the absence of such modification, sperm–egg binding is inhibited (Talansky 1992). This can be demonstrated by incubating capacitated sperm with oocytes, in the presence of high concentrations of the surface glycoproteins isolated from uncapacitated sperm, when egg–sperm binding does not occur. These glycoproteins are called 'decapacitation factors' (Yanagimachi 1988).

The binding of the sperm with the zona pellucida is a tenacious and specific contact (which occurs after an initial loose, reversible, non-specific attachment). Oocyte maturity is important in this process, mature oocytes showing increased binding as compared with immature or atretic ones.

After binding of the sperm to the oocyte, another process takes place called the sperm acrosome reaction. This involves the release of the contents of the acrosome and the exposure of the inner acrosomal membrane, to facilitate penetration of the zona pellucida by the sperm (Huang and Yanagimachi 1985).

Micromanipulation of oocytes (by techniques such as sub-zonal sperm insertion and partial zona dissection) is rapidly gaining ground as research in this field advances. It is known, for example, that sperm that are still acrosome-intact can undergo spontaneous acrosome reaction after micromanipulation procedures. Fertilisation has been demonstrated in human oocytes after subzonal insertion of immotile sperm from a male with Kartagener's syndrome (Bongso *et al.* 1989). Micromanipulation procedures are now being applied increasingly for various forms of severe male factor infertility (Cohen *et al.* 1991).

REFERENCES

Bongso, T.A., Sathananthan, A.H., Wong, P.C. *et al.* (1989) Human fertilization by micro-injection of immotile spermatozoa. *Hum Reprod* **4**, 175-9

Cohen, J., Alikani, M., Malter, H.E. *et al.* (1991) Partial zona dissection or subzonal sperm insertion: microsurgical fertilization alternatives based on evaluation of sperm and embryo morphology. *Fertil Steril* **56**, 696-706

Huang, T.T.F. and Yanagimachi, R. (1985) Inner acrosomal membrane of mammalian spermatozoa: its properties and possible functions in fertilization. *Am J Anat* **174**, 249-68

Lambert, H., Overstreet, J.W., Morales, P. *et al.* (1985) Sperm capacitation in the human female reproductive tract. *Fertil Steril* **43**, 325-7

Plachot, M., Junca, A.M., Mandlebaum, J. *et al.* (1985) Timing of *in-vitro* fertilization of cumulus-free and cumulus-enclosed oocytes. *Hum Reprod* **1**, 237-42

Plachot, M. and Mandelbaum, J. (1990) 'Oocyte maturation, fertilization and embryonic growth *in vitro*' in R.G. Edwards (Ed.) *Assisted Human Reproduction*, pp. 675-94. Edinburgh: Churchill Livingstone

Talansky, B.E. (1992) 'Fertilization and early embryonic development in the human' in J. Cohen *et al.* (Eds) *Micromanipulation of Human Gametes and Embryos*, pp. 84-112. New York: Raven Press

Yanagimachi, R. (1988) 'Mammalian fertilization' in E. Knobil *et al.* (Eds) *The Physiology of Reproduction*, pp. 135-85. New York: Raven Press

83   Which of the following statements regarding abnormal vaginal bleeding are correct?

A) Less than 1% of endometrial adenocarcinomas occur in women under 35.	TRUE
B) Approximately 6% of endometrial adenocarcinomas occur in women under 45.	TRUE
C) Dilatation and curettage alone will miss 10% of endometrial pathology.	TRUE
D) Dilatation and curettage has been shown to have a greater therapeutic effect than previously thought.	FALSE
E) Pipelle de Cornier endometrial sampling not only avoids general anaesthesia but is as accurate as outpatient hysteroscopy.	FALSE

COMMENTS

Dilatation and curettage is almost certainly used in the UK (Coulter *et al.* 1993). It is therapeutically ineffective and diagnostically inaccurate (Grimes 1982). Simple outpatient techniques of endometrial sampling are well justified as their accuracy approaches that of dilatation and curettage but avoids the disruption and risk of general anaesthesia (Stovall *et al.* 1991). Dilatation and curettage misses 10% of endometrial pathology (including benign and malignant) (Word *et al.* 1958). Pathology such as endometrial polyps and fibroids may be missed. However, the prime aim of such sampling is to exclude endometrial adenocarcinoma in women between the ages of 35 and 50. Less than 1% of such malignancies occur in women under 35 and about 6% in women below 45 (Pettersson 1990).

REFERENCES

Coulter, A., Klassen, A., MacKenzie, I.Z. *et al.* (1993) Diagnostic dilatation and curettage: is it used appropriately? *BMJ* **306**, 236-9

Grimes, D.A. (1982) Diagnostic dilatation and curettage. *Am J Obstet Gynecol* **142**, 1-6

Pettersson, F. (1990) Annual report on the results of treatment in gynaecological cancer. *Int J Gynaecol Obstet* **97**, 139

Stovall, T., Ling, F. and Morgan, P. (1991) A prospective randomised comparison of the Pipelle endometrial sampling device with the Novak curette. *Am J Obstet Gynecol* **165**, 1287-9

Word, B., Gravlee, L.C. and Wideman, G.L. (1958) The fallacy of simple uterine curettage. *Obstet Gynecol* **12**, 642-7

84 In the management of subfertility:

A) The most common site for tubal damage is the end of the tube.   TRUE

B) Surgery for occlusion of the proximal end of the tube is less successful than that for the distal end.   FALSE

C) Treatment of mild endometriosis is effective in increasing fertility.   FALSE

D) Medical treatment for ovulatory dysfunction caused by hyperprolactinaemia or hypothalamic amenorrhoea may restore fertility to near normal levels.   TRUE

E) Controlled trials have shown drugs to be ineffective in the management of idiopathic male subfertility.   TRUE

COMMENTS

Eighty per cent of cases of tubal damage involve the distal end of the tube. Surgery results in 20-30% success rates, depending on severity (Marana and Quagliarello 1988). Surgery for occlusion of the proximal end is more successful, with rates of 40-60% reported (Patton *et al.* 1987). The ectopic pregnancy rate for distal tube surgery is up to 25%, whereas for proximal tubal surgery is usually less than 10%.

The relationship between endometriosis and subfertility is unclear. Many women with endometriosis conceive successfully without intervention and controlled trials have not shown an improved pregnancy rate with treatment of the endometriosis (Badawy *et al.* 1988).

Treatment of ovulatory dysfunction, particularly bromocriptine or similar agents for hyperprolactinaemia and gonadotrophins for hypothalamic amenorrhoea are extremely effective (Hull *et al.* 1979). Various empirical treatments have been used to treat idiopathic male subfertility, but controlled trials have shown these to be ineffective (World Health Organisation 1989).

REFERENCES

Badawy, S.Z., Elbakry, M.M., Samuel, F. *et al.* (1988) Cumulative pregnancy rates in infertile women with endometriosis. *J Reprod Med* 757-60

Hull, M.G.R., Savage, P.E. and Jacobs, H.S. (1979) Investigation and treatment of amenorrhoea resulting in normal fertility. *BMJ* 1257-61

Marana, R. and Quagliarello, J. (1988) Proximal tubal occlusion: microsurgery versus IVF – a review. *Int J Fertil* **33**, 338-40

Patton, P.E., Williams, T.J. and Coulam, C.B. (1987) Microsurgical reconstruction of the proximal oviduct. *Fertil Steril* **47**, 35-9

World Health Organisation (1989) WHO Task Force on the diagnosis and treatment of infertility. Mesterolone and idiopathic male infertility: a double-blind study. *Int J Androl* **12**, 254-64

85 With regard to colposcopy, which of the following statements are correct?

A) 0.3% acetic acid is used to differentiate between CIN and the normal transformation zone. FALSE

B) Increased mucus production at mid cycle makes this an inappropriate time to examine the endocervix. FALSE

C) The combination of aceto white and mosaic is diagnostic of glandular epithelial neoplasia. FALSE

D) Tissue necrosis after treatment with the 30 watt CO_2 laser extends 4 mm beyond the limit of visible tissue destruction. FALSE

E) Patients who have CIN3 are more likely to have anal and intraepithelial neoplasia than are women with normal cervices. TRUE

COMMENTS

Three per cent or 5% acetic acid is used to differentiate between CIN and the transformation zone. Because the cervix everts and opens slightly at mid cycle and ovulatory mucus is transparent, the endocervical canal is more easily visualised.

Aceto white and mosaic are colposcopic abnormalities seen in the transformation zone and indicate squamous intraepithelial neoplasia. The colposcopic appearances of glandular intraepithelial neoplasia are so variable that the diagnosis cannot be made with confidence from the colposcopic appearance.

With the CO_2 laser, tissue destruction does not extend to two or three cells beyond the region of visible destruction.

One common aetiological factor shared by invasive carcinomas of the ano-genital epithelium is HPV type 16 and HPV infection of one area of ano-genital epithelium can be rapidly followed by infection of adjacent areas, making them susceptible to neoplastic change. One survey of 152 women with CIN3 found anal intraepithelial neoplasia in 7% of those whose only other lesion was of the cervix but in 57% of those where there was CIN3 plus intraepithelial neoplasia of the vulva and/or vagina. The control group of 50 women contained no cases of anal intraepithelial neoplasia (Schofield et al. 1992).

REFERENCE

Schofield, J.H., Hickson, W.G.E., Smith, J.H.F. et al. (1992) Anal intraepithelial neoplasia: part of a multifocal disease process. *Lancet* **240**, 1271-3

86 In women with laparoscopically proven endometriosis:

A) Pain relates to prostaglandin F production by the lesions. **TRUE**
B) The rate of spontaneous abortion is increased. **TRUE**
C) Danazol increases sex hormone binding globulin (SHBG) production. **FALSE**
D) Danazol has no proven effect on fertility. **TRUE**
E) GnRH analogues are more effective than danazol in reducing pelvic pain and dysmenorrhoea. **FALSE**

COMMENTS

Pain, particularly dysmenorrhoea, is a common symptom of endometriosis. One striking feature of the disease is a poor correlation between the severity of the disease and the degree of pain experienced by the patient. It has been shown, however, that endometriotic implants are capable of producing prostaglandin (Ylikorkala and Viinikka 1983) and that pain scores relate to the production of PGF by these tissues. The data for prostaglandin production by peritoneal fluid in women with endometriosis have shown inconsistent results. This may be a reflection on the pitfalls in prostaglandin assays (Kelly 1985).

Endometriosis has an association with both infertility and an increased spontaneous abortion rate (Sutton 1990; Malinak and Wheeler 1986).

Danazol, an isoxazole derivative of 17-ethynyl testosterone inhibits ovarian and adrenal steroidogenesis. It decreases SHBG production thereby increasing free testosterone levels accounting for the androgenic side-effects. Danazol also produces reversible effects on lipoproteins including elevation of low-density lipoproteins and reduction of high-density lipoproteins and cholesterol (Fahraeus et al. 1984). There is some evidence that endometriosis is an autoimmune disease and the immunosuppressive qualities of danazol may contribute to its effectiveness (Rock and Moutos 1992).

The GnRH analogues do not produce significant effects on lipoprotein levels but they do produce a small but significant decrease in trabecular bone mineral content. There are no significant differences in the alleviation of symptoms between danazol and the GnRH analogues.

REFERENCES

Fahraeus, L., Larsson-Cohn, U., Ljunberg, S. et al. (1984) Profound alterations of the lipoprotein metabolism during danazol treatment in pre-menopausal women. *Fertil Steril* **42**, 52-7

Kelly, R.W. (1985) Prostaglandin measurement: potential and limitations. *Prostaglandin Perspectives* **2**, 3-4

Malinak, L.R. and Wheeler, J.M. (1986) Association of endometriosis with spontaneous abortion: prognosis for pregnancy and risk of occurrence. *Semin Reprod Endocrinol* **3**, 361-9

Rock, J.A. and Moutos, D.M. (1992) Endometriosis: the present and the future – an overview of treatment options. *Br J Obstet Gynaecol* **99** (Suppl) 1-4

Sutton, C. (1990) 'The treatment of endometriosis' in J. Studd (Ed.) *Progress in Obstetrics and Gynaecology*, **8**, pp. 251-71. Edinburgh: Churchill Livingstone

Ylikorkala, V. and Viinikka, L. (1983) Prostaglandins and endometriosis. *Acta Obstet Gynaecol Scand* **113** (Suppl), 105-7

87 Combined oestrogen progesterone hormone replacement therapy:

A) Should be offered to a 40-year-old woman undergoing a premature menopause. TRUE
B) Should be offered to a 45-year-old woman undergoing total abdominal hysterectomy and bilateral salpingo-oophorectomy (TAH and BSO) for menorrhagia. FALSE
C) Is contraindicated after radiotherapy for cervical carcinoma. FALSE
D) Is contraindicated in a woman with a first-degree relative with coronary artery disease. FALSE
E) Is contraindicated after TAH and BSO for extensive pelvic endometriosis. FALSE

COMMENTS

Postmenopausal HRT is indicated for the treatment of the symptoms of oestrogen deficiency and prevention of long-term complications such as osteoporosis and cardiovascular disease (Jacobs and Loeffler 1992).

The effectiveness of oestrogen therapy in increasing calcium absorption, reducing calcium excretion and reducing the incidence of fractures due to osteoporosis is well proven. Women who have an early menopause, who are thin, who smoke or who have a family history of osteoporosis are at particular risk, and should be offered HRT. Combined therapy with oestrogen and progesterone should be offered if the uterus is intact, as the use of unopposed oestrogen increases the risk of endometrial cancer (Henderson 1989).

The effectiveness of oestrogen and progesterone therapy in the prevention of cardiovascular disease is more controversial, partly due to the unreasonable comparison of HRT to the oral contraceptive pill. There is good evidence that unopposed oestrogen therapy in doses suitable for replacement treatment reduces the risk of cardiovascular disease by 40% (reviewed by Bush and Miller-Bass 1991). There is some evidence that the addition of progestogens to oestrogen therapy may reverse the favourable effects of the oestrogens on lipids and lipoproteins (Notelovitz, 1989). At present it is not known whether opposed oestrogen therapy attenuates the reduction in cardiovascular disease seen with unopposed oestrogens. It is generally agreed, however, that after hysterectomy oestrogen therapy alone should be offered (Jacobs and Loeffler 1992). There is evidence that oestrogens are involved in the aetiology of breast and endometrial cancer, but not cervical or ovarian carcinoma (Studd and Baber 1992). Treatment should not therefore be denied to women who have been treated for cervical carcinoma.

Radical pelvic surgery for endometriosis is the final resort in treatment to control symptoms of intractable pain when fertility is no longer an issue. Women who have undergone bilateral oophorectomy will be rendered hypoestrogenic. Progesterones may be effective in treating the residual endometriosis and there is evidence that the dose of oestrogen in HRT is not sufficient to stimulate the disease (Henderson and Studd 1991).

REFERENCES

Bush, T.L. and Miller-Bass, K. (1991) Oestrogen therapy and cardiovascular disease: do the benefits outweigh the risk? *Baillière's Clin Obstet Gynaecol* 4: 5, 889-913

Henderson, B.E. (1989) The cancer question: an overview of recent epidemiologic and retrospective data. *Am J Obstet Gynecol* **161**, 1859-63

Henderson, A.S.F. and Studd, J.W.W. (1991) 'The role of definitive surgery and hormone replacement therapy in the treatment of endometriosis' in E.J. Thomas and J.A. Rock (Eds) *Modern Approaches to Endometriosis*, pp. 275-90. London: Kluwer Academic

Jacobs, H.S. and Loeffler, F.E. (1992) Postmenopausal hormone replacement therapy. *BMJ* **305**, 1403-8

Notelovitz, M. (1989) Oestrogen replacement therapy: indications, contra-indications and agent selection. *Am J Obstet Gynecol* **161** 1832-41

Studd, J.W.W. and Baber, J. (1992) 'The menopause' in E.W. Shaw, W.P. Soutter and S.L. Stanton (Eds) *Gynaecology*, pp. 341-54. Edinburgh: Churchill Livingstone

88 **With regard to a woman who has one close relative with ovarian cancer which of the following statements are correct?**

A) She is at no increased risk of developing the disease herself.	FALSE
B) She is more at risk of developing either breast, colon or stomach cancer.	TRUE
C) She should be enrolled in the UKCCR Familial Ovarian Cancer Study.	FALSE
D) She should be offered annual screening by ultrasound scan.	FALSE
E) She should be offered prophylactic oophorectomy if childbearing is complete.	FALSE

COMMENTS

Women who have only one close relative with ovarian cancer are, on current estimates, at slightly increased risk of developing the disease themselves. Compared with the population as a whole the risk is increased about three-fold. This translates as a 1:40 chance of death from ovarian cancer by age 70.

There is evidence that other cancers, such as breast, colon, stomach, are slightly more frequent in the relatives of ovarian cancer patients and in some families there appears to be an increased risk of breast and ovarian cancer of colo-rectal and ovarian cancer together.

Only women who have two or more close relatives with ovarian cancer (whether still living or dead) or who themselves have ovarian cancer and also an affected close relative should be registered with the UKCCR Familial Ovarian Cancer Study at the CRC Human Cancer Genetics Research Group, Cambridge.

Screening for ovarian cancer is of unproven benefit at present. Nevertheless, in families with two or more cases of epithelial ovarian cancer annual screening by pelvic and general examination with abdominal or vaginal ultrasound scan is recommended. If the ultrasound is positive, a second line screening test of greater specificity (colour Doppler ovarian blood-flow measurement) is recommended before surgical exploration.

The decision for prophylactic oophorectomy is an individual one for each patient and even in high-risk families it is usually reasonable to wait until childbearing is complete. Because some ovarian cancers seem to arise primarily at extra-ovarian sites, oophorectomy may provide incomplete protection.

APPROPRIATE READING

Lynch, H.T., Albano, W.A. Lynch, J.F *et al.* (1982) Surveillance and management of patients at high risk for ovarian cancer. *Obstet Gynecol* **59**, 589-96

Ponder, B.A.J., Easton, D.F. and Peto, J. (1990) 'Risk of ovarian cancer associated with a family history: preliminary report of the OPCS study' in F. Sharp, W.P. Mason and R.E. Leake (Eds) *Ovarian Cancer*, pp. 3-6. London: Chapman and Hall

Schildkraut, J.M. and Thompson, W.D. (1988) Familial ovarian cancer: a population-based case control study. *Am J Epidemiol* **128**, 456-66

89 Which of the following statements regarding transvaginal scans are correct?

A) A full bladder helps to obtain a better definition during a transvaginal scan.   FALSE

B) An endometrial thickness of >5 mm is indicative of an endometrial neoplasm in
     postmenopausal women.   FALSE

C) They will reliably detect ovarian neoplasms.   FALSE

D) They can reliably diagnose abdominal wall defects at <10 weeks' gestation.   FALSE

E) They are dangerous in the presence of a placenta praevia.   FALSE

COMMENTS

Transvaginal scans are ideal for use in gynaecology and early obstetric practice. In conventional transabdominal scanning of the pelvis, a full bladdder is essential in order to displace bowel and to create a window through which the uterus and its contents can be visualised. This is time-consuming and uncomfortable for the patient. Despite filling the bladder the pelvic structures are still some way from the transducer, and in obese patients the view is far from ideal. In transvaginal scanning, the transducer is placed inside the vagina in close proximity to the structures to be scanned. Bowel and fat does not intervene and a much clearer view may be obtained. A full bladder is not needed and may in fact hinder the examination by displacing structures from the near field of view.

Because of the much enhanced view the structure of the ovaries and uterus is clearly seen and carcinomas of the endometrium and ovary can be clearly visualised. One important proviso must be recognised: because of the limited depth of penetration, large masses pushed out of the pelvis may be missed altogether, and if the clinical examination suggests this, or the ovaries are not seen, a transabdominal scan should be performed.

Various studies have examined the thickness of the endometrium in postmenopausal women. A measurement of <5 mm appears to indicate a normal atrophic endometrium, with a sensitivity of 100% and 96% specificity. Between 5 mm and 8 mm very few carcinomas appear to be found, but proliferative endometrium, hyperplasia polyps, etc. are detected. Most carcinomas have been detected at >8 mm, and when symptomatic with PMB one study found a mean thickness of 20 mm.

TV scans are very useful in early pregnancy to determine viability etc. Whilst many anomalies have been detected at <10 weeks, care must be exercised as appearances which are abnormal during the second trimester may be a normal part of development in early pregnancy, e.g. exomphalos.

Traditionally, vaginal examination has been contraindicated in women with an antepartum haemorrhage thought to be due to a placenta praevia. Instead a speculum examination has been recommended. Some worry about inserting an ultrasound probe into the vagina in such circumstances, but as this need not touch the cervix or lower segment this appears irrational. Several studies have shown the safety and efficacy of transvaginal scans in these circumstances, giving a very good view of the internal os and its relation to the placenta whether anterior or posterior and obscured by the fetal head.

APPROPRIATE READING

Dewbury, K., Meire, H. and Cosgrove, D. (Eds) (1992) *Ultrasound in Obstetrics and Gynaecology*. Edinburgh: Churchill Livingstone

90 In accordance with regulations in the Human Fertilisation and Embryology Act 1990 and the Code of Practice outlined by the Human Fertilisation and Embryology Authority (HFEA), which of the following apply?

A) In any one IVF cycle no more than five embryos are to be replaced.   FALSE
B) Sperm may be cryopreserved for an indefinite period.   FALSE
C) Only an upper age limit is imposed on donors of sperm and oocytes.   FALSE
D) A child born from the use of donor sperm is illegitimate.   FALSE
E) Research may not be carried out on embryos after the development of the primitive streak.   TRUE

COMMENTS

Prior to the Human Fertilisation and Embryology Act 1990 there had been no legislation regarding the use and storage of human embryos. The Voluntary Licensing Authority set up in 1985, which was superseded by the Interim Licensing Authority (1989), recommended that no more than three embryos, or four in exceptional circumstances, be placed into a woman in any one treatment cycle. Before this there was no limit to the number of embryos which could be replaced. The Human Fertilisation and Embryology Authority's Code of Practice (7.9) states that no more than three embryos are to be replaced in any one treatment cycle.

Any man consenting to the storage of his sperm should be made aware that the maximum period of storage is ten years (HF&E Act, Section 14.3). However, he can specify the period of storage if this is to be less than the statutory period (ibid. Section 14.5(A)), and he also needs to state what is to be done with the sperm should he die or become incapable of varying or revoking his consent (ibid. Schedule 3.2(2)).

The Human Fertilisation and Embryology Authority (HFEA) places both upper and lower age limits on the donors of gametes. The *Code of Practice* (3.33; 3.34) states that gametes should not be taken for the treatment of others from female donors over the age of 35, unless there are exceptional circumstances. It also precludes the use of gametes taken from anyone under 18 in the treatment of others (3.35).

Prior to the HF&E Act any child born following the use of donor sperm, even though the husband or partner had agreed to the treatment, was illegitimate. Under the Act, a woman's husband will be the legal father of a child born as a result of treatment using donated sperm unless they are judicially separated or he can prove that he did not consent to the treatment. If a woman is treated with a male partner using donated sperm, and she is unmarried or judicially separated or her husband does not consent to the treatment, her male partner will be the legal father of any resulting child (HFEA *Code of Practice* 5.7; 5.8. HF&E Act, Section 28).

All research which involves the creation, keeping or using of human embryos outside the body must be licensed by the Human Fertilisation and Embryology Authority and the keeping or using of an embryo after the appearance of the primitive streak or 14 days post-fertilisation is prohibited by law (HF&E Act, Section 3; 3(a)).

REFERENCES

Human Fertilisation and Embryology (HF&E) Act, 1990

Human Fertilisation and Embryology Authority (1993) *Code of Practice* (revised ed.). London HFEA

91 The tumour marker CA125:

A) Is raised in more than 80% of ovarian cancer.   TRUE
B) Is a specific ovarian tumour marker.   FALSE
C) Is useful in screening for ovarian cancer.   FALSE
D) Correlates with the disease course in 90% of ovarian cancer.   TRUE
E) Can be used to replace second-look laparotomy.   FALSE

COMMENTS

CA125 is raised in pancreatic cancer, breast, lung and colorectal cancers. CA125 is not specific enough for screening of ovarian cancer. It is raised in endometriosis, pelvic inflammatory disease and peritonitis. There is a false positive rate of 0.6% in postmenopausal women.

Residual tumours were found in 40% of patients with normal CA125 before second look laparotomy (Berek *et al.* 1986).

REFERENCE

Berek, J.S., Knapp, R.C., Malkasian, G.D. *et al.* (1986) CA125 serum levels correlated with second-look operations among ovarian cancer patients. *Obstet Gynecol* **67**, 685-9

APPROPRIATE READING

Niloff, J.M., Knapp, R.C., Schaetzl, E. *et al.* (1984) CA125 antigen levels in obstetric and gynecologic patients. *Obstet Gynecol* **64**, 703-7

Zurawski, V.R., Briderick, S.F., Pickens, P. *et al.* (1987) Serum CA125 levels in a large group of non-hospitalized women: relevance for the early detection of ovarian cancer. *Obstet Gynecol* **69**, 606-11

92 In the investigation and management of infertility:

A) Sonographic hydrotubation and colour Doppler studies of tubal patency are less effective than hysterosalpingography in the diagnosis of tubal patency. FALSE
B) Effective treatment of endometriosis doubles the chances of conception. FALSE
C) Smoking does not affect the outcome of ovulation induction. FALSE
D) Assisted conception techniques (in vitro fertilisation, gamete intra-fallopian transfer, intrauterine insemination and superovulation) carry a 50% chance of pregnancy compared with fertile couples in the long term. FALSE
E) Down-regulation (desensitisation) of the pituitary gland before ovulation induction does not increase the conception rate in assisted conception techniques. FALSE

COMMENTS

A study by Mitri et al. (1991) shows that vaginal sonographic hydrotubation is as effective as hysterosalpingography (HSG) in 70-80% of cases, and in the remainder is likely to be superior, particularly in the demonstration of hydrosalpinges with cornual blockage, coexistent ovarian pathology and the presence of subserous and intramural fibroids. The risk of reaction to the contrast medium is removed, as is concern regarding gonadal irritation. However, pregnancy must still be excluded prior to the procedure, as fluid is being instilled into the endometrial cavity. Similarly, Stern et al. (1992) showed that colour Doppler studies of tubal patency correlated with laparoscopic dye hydrotubation in 81% of patients compared with 60% correlation between HSG and dye hydrotubation. However, the HSG gives information about the internal structure of the tubes, which neither of the two sonographic techniques can provide.

Hull et al. (1987) showed that neither treatment with progestational agents or danazol is superior to expectant management in increasing conception rates in infertile patients with endometriosis.

Van Voorhis et al. (1992) showed that smokers in an assisted reproduction group had lower serum oestradiol levels, fewer follicles, fewer oocytes retrieved and fewer embryos per cycle than non-smokers. This backed up previous studies by Barbieri et al. (1986) which showed inhibition of granulosa cell aromatase enzyme activity in vitro, and by Harrison et al. (1990) and Elenbogen et al. (1991) showing that smokers have reduced ovarian responsiveness in terms of longer stimulations with more ampoules of gonadotrophins being required. Interestingly, a study on fertilisation rates in in-vitro patients in whom a nicotine metabolite was sought in aspirated ovarian follicular fluid showed a significantly lower fertilisation rate when the metabolite was detectable than when absent (70% versus 57%) (Rosevear et al. 1992).

A study by Hull et al. (1992) showed that cumulative conception rate in assisted conception techniques, if couples persist in treatment, is at least as good as for fertile couples, except for women over 40 and men with sperm dysfunction.

A meta-analysis of ten studies of the use of down-regulation in assisted conception shows that this doubles the conception rates and halves the number of abandoned cycles (Hughes et al. 1992).

REFERENCES

Barbieri, R.L., McShane, P.M. and Ryan, K.J. (1986) Constituents of cigarette smoke inhibit human granulosa cell aromatose. *Fertil Steril* **46**, 232-6

Elenbogen, A., Lipitz, S., Mashiach, S. et al. (1991) The effect of smoking on the outcome of in vitro fertilisation – embryo transfer. *Hum Reprod* **6**, 242-4

Harrison, K.L., Breen, T.M. and Hennessey, J.F. (1990) The effect of patient smoking habit on the outcome of IVF GIFT treatment. *Aust NZ J Obstet Gynaecol* **30**, 340-2

Hughes, E.G., Fedorkow, D.M., Daya, S. et al. (1992) The routine use of gonadotrophin-releasing hormone agonists prior to in vitro fertilisation and gamete intrafallopian transfers, a meta-analysis of randomised control trials. *Fertil Steril* **58**, 888-96

Hull, M.E., Moghissi, K.S., Magyar, D.F. et al. (1987) Comparison of different treatment modalities of endometriosis in infertile women. *Fertil Steril*, **47**, 40-4

Hull, M.G.R., Eddowes, H.A., Fahy, U. et al. (1992) Expectations of assisted conception for infertility. *BMJ* **304**, 1465-9

Mitri, F.F., Andronikou, A.D., Perpinyal, S. *et al.* (1991) A clinical comparison of sonographic hydrotubation and hysterosalpingography. *Br J Obstet Gynaecol* **98**, 1031-6

Rosevear, S.K., Holt, D.W., Lee, T.D. *et al.* (1992) Smoking and decreased fertilisation rates *in vitro*. *Lancet* **340**, 1195-6

Stern, J., Peters, A.J. and Coulam, C.B. (1992) Color Doppler ultrasonography assessment of tubal patency: a comparison with traditional techniques. *Fertil Steril* **58**, 897-901

Van Voorhis, B.J., Syrop, C.H., Hammitt, D.J. *et al.* (1992) Effects of smoking on ovulation induction for assisted reproductive techniques. *Fertil Steril* **58**, 981-5

93 Hysteroscopy:

A) Detects intrauterine pathology in up to 85% of patients with abnormal uterine bleeding.   TRUE

B) Has higher diagnostic accuracy than hysterosalpingography.   TRUE

C) Does not require prior dilatation of the cervix.   FALSE

D) Is essential in women under 35 years to exclude endometrial carcinoma as a cause of abnormal bleeding.   FALSE

E) Is contraindicated in the presence of pelvic sepsis.   TRUE

COMMENTS

Hysteroscopy is endoscopic inspection of the uterine cavity through the cervix. It has high diagnostic accuracy in the investigation of abnormal uterine bleeding (Mencaglia *et al.* 1987). In premenopausal women polyps, submucous fibroids and endometrial hyperplasia are most common. Hysteroscopy is better at detecting abnormalities than hysterosalpingography, and is an important investigation in the management of infertility and recurrent miscarriage.

The patient is placed in the modified lithotomy position, and after cleansing the cervical os is dilated to Hegar size 6 or 7.

Abnormal premenopausal bleeding is very rarely due to endometrial carcinoma (Hammond *et al.* 1989). Less than 1% of adenocarcinomas of the endometrium occur in women under 35 and only 6% occur in women up to the age of 45 (Patterson 1990). Pelvic infection, vaginal infection and cervicitis should all be adequately treated before hysteroscopy (Bates and Lewis 1993).

REFERENCES

Bates, S.A. and Lewis, B.V. (1993) Hysteroscopy and endometrial ablation. *Hosp Update* **19**, 39-44

Hammond, R., Oppenheimer, L. and Saunders, P. (1989) Diagnostic role of dilatation and curettage in the management of abnormal premenopausal bleeding. *Br J Obstet Gynaecol* **96**, 496-7

Mencaglia, L., Perino, A. and Hamon, J. (1987) Hysteroscopy on perimenopausal women with abnormal uterine bleeding. *J Reprod Med* **32**, 577-9

Patterson, F. (1990) Annual report on the results of treatment in gynaecological cancer. *Int J Gynaecol Obstet* **21**, 139

94 **In anorexia nervosa, the following statements are correct:**

A)	The onset is between ages 30 and 40.	FALSE
B)	The weight is 25% below normal for age and weight.	TRUE
C)	Diarrhoea is a common symptom.	FALSE
D)	There are persistently low levels of FSH and LH.	TRUE
E)	Plasma cortisol levels are elevated.	TRUE

COMMENTS

Anorexia nervosa occurs almost exclusively in young, white, middle to upper social class females under the age of 25. The families of anorexics are success-achievement-appearance orientated. The pattern usually starts with a voluntary diet to control weight. Excessive physical activity can be the earliest sign. Basically, an eating disorder is a method being utilised to solve a psychological dilemma. Weight loss of 25% or weight 15% below normal for age and height is indicative.

Besides amenorrhoea, constipation is a common symptom, often severe and accompanied by abdominal pain. Endocrine studies show low levels of FSH and LH; normal prolactin; TSH and T4 are normal but T3 levels are low. Cortisol levels are elevated due to decreased clearance in the face of a normal production rate.

APPROPRIATE READING

Speroff, L., Glass, R.H. and Kase, N.G. (1994) 'Anorexia nervosa' in *Clinical Gynecologic Endocrinology and Infertility* (5th ed.), pp. 435-8. Baltimore: Williams and Wilkins

95 In the use of diathermy, the following apply:

A) A coagulating waveform consists of a continuous radio frequency sinewave.	FALSE
B) A cut waveform has a lower peak voltage than a coagulating waveform.	TRUE
C) In a liquid medium, the coagulation waveform causes fewer bubbles than a cut waveform.	FALSE
D) Coagulation requires contact between the electrode and tissue.	FALSE
E) Cutting diathermy will desiccate tissue.	TRUE

COMMENTS

The use of diathermy has expanded greatly in gynaecological surgery with the growth of endometrial ablation/resection and operative laparoscopy. This is not helped by differing authors suggesting different waveforms and voltages. To interpret these papers safely and to achieve the best and safest results the operator should have some knowledge of the properties of radio-frequency waves used in surgical diathermy. All surgical diathermy machines generate a sinusoidal waveform which may be continuous or modulated/damped. Cutting diathermy employs a constant flow of energy in a continuous waveform. As the energy flow is constant, to achieve a certain power requires a lower peak voltage. Coagulation waveforms are interrupted, intermittent or damped, and require higher peak voltages to achieve a given power output. A blended current combines a continuous waveform with superimposed pulses. With a small active electrode, the current density is high, and will heat the tissue in contact with it. A burn will also occur if the return electrode is not of sufficient size for the same reason. As the current follows the path of least resistance to the return electrode, burns may occur when current is unintentionally concentrated into a small area, of importance in laparoscopic surgery where the current may jump small gaps of 1-2 mm. The use of the lowest possible voltage to achieve the required result is therefore a good principle in laparoscopic surgery. Bipolar diathermy uses the indulated jaws of forceps as active and return electrodes to coagulate tissue. It is inherently safer, but of less practical application in many circumstances.

Coagulation can be divided into desiccation and fulguration (spray). The former occurs when moist tissue touches the electrode, heat being dispersed more widely by the bursts of energy, the cells being dehydrated and killed. To be effective the electrode must be kept clean. In fulguration the current jumps across small air/fluid gaps or desiccated tissue with a high resistance and produces charring and necrosis over a wider but shallower area than that obtained with desiccation. Current flow ceases when all tissue in reach of the sparking has been coagulated and the resistance becomes too high.

Current flow in fulguration is around one-fifth of that in desiccation. Coagulation diathermy electrodes tend to have a relatively large contact area compared with cutting diathermy electrodes. When using cutting diathermy, the contact area is small in order to concentrate the constant current over a small area. This causes the cells to explode as the water content flashes to steam, and creates a cut rather than necrosis. Contact is not necessary, and pressure of the electrode on the tissue may in fact make the cut less easy. When a cutting current is applied to a larger electrode cutting does not occur easily. Desiccation will occur, but fulguration will not. In a fluid medium more bubbles are generated in coagulation mode than cutting.

APPROPRIATE READING

Soderstrom, R.M. (1992) Electricity inside the uterus. *Clin Obstet Gynecol* **35**: 2, 262-9

Instruction Manual for the Valleylab Force 2 Electrosurgical Generator. (Obtainable from Valleylab (UK) Ltd, Unit 5, Royal London Estate, 29-35 North Acton Road, London NW10 6PE.)

96   Following treatment of cervical intraepithelial neoplasia (CIN):

A) There is a high incidence of cervical stenosis.   FALSE
B) Subsequent fertility is compromised.   FALSE
C) There is an increased incidence of mid-trimester abortion in a future pregnancy
   after knife cone biopsy.   TRUE
D) By destructive techniques, the incidence of preterm labour is increased in a
   subsequent pregnancy.   FALSE
E) By destructive techniques, the incidence of Caesarean section is increased in a
   subsequent pregnancy.   FALSE

COMMENTS

Luesley *et al.* (1985) reported symptomatic cervical stenosis in 8% of 915 patients following cone biopsy; it does not appear to be a problem following destructive treatment techniques. Although there are a number of potential causes of infertility after treatment of CIN, there are no reports of decreased fertility in such patients (Hammond and Edmonds 1990). Lieman *et al.* (1980) reported an incidence of mid-trimester abortion of 15% in 88 pregnancies in 77 women following cervical conisation. There does not appear to be any increased risk in a subsequent pregnancy following destructive treatments for cervical intraepithelial neoplasia.

REFERENCES

Hammond, R.H. and Edmonds, D.K. (1990) Does treatment for cervical intraepithelial neoplasia affect fertility and pregnancy? *BMJ* **301**, 1344-5

Lieman, G., Harrison, N.A., Rubin, A. (1980) Pregnancy following conisation of the cervix: complications related to cone size. *Am J Obstet Gynecol* **136**, 14-18

Luesley, D.M., McCrum, A., Terry, P.B. *et al.* (1985) Complications of cone biopsy related to the dimensions of the cone and the influence of prior colposcopic assessment. *Br J Obstet Gynaecol* **92**, 158-64

97 Borderline epithelial ovarian tumours:

A) Have a 95% plus five-year survival rate in Stage I disease.	TRUE
B) Represent approximately 12% of all epithelial ovarian neoplasms.	TRUE
C) May have a high bilateral incidence.	TRUE
D) Should be treated by TAH, BSO and adjuvent therapy.	FALSE
E) Have a 5% recurrence rate in conservatively managed Stage I disease.	FALSE

COMMENTS

A distinct borderline category of epithelial ovarian tumours was introduced by FIGO in 1961 and was approved by WHO in 1973. Their features consist of epithelial cell stratification, increased mitotic activity, nuclear abnormalities and cytologically atypical cells without invasion of the adjacent stroma. Five-year survival rates in excess of 95% are recorded for Stage I borderline tumours (Piver 1987). The incidence of borderline tumours as a proportion of all ovarian epithelial tumours is reported as between 9% and 16% (Nation and Kreport 1986), and bilaterality rates of up to 40% have been reported (Yoonessi *et al.* 1988). The issue of conservative treatment has been controversial (Ayhan *et al.* 1991) and if future fertility is not a concern TAH and BSO is the safest course but there would seem to be insufficient evidence to suggest the addition of adjuvent therapy. A recurrence rate of 15% for conservatively managed Stage I disease has been reported (Tazelaar *et al.* 1985) and 40% for treatment by cystectomy alone (Chambers *et al.* 1988).

REFERENCES

Ayhan, A., Akarin, R., Develioglu, O. *et al.* (1991) Borderline epithelial ovarian tumours. *Aust NZ J Obstet Gynaecol* **31**, 174-6

Chambers, J.T., Merino, M.J., Kohorn, E.L. (1988) Borderline ovarian tumours. *Am J Obstet Gynecol* **159**, 1088-94

Nation, J.G. and Kreport, G.V. (1986) Ovarian carcinoma of low malignant potential: staging and treatment. *Am J Obstet Gynecol* **154** 290-3

Piver, M.S. (Ed.) (1987) 'Progress and treatment of borderline ovarian tumors' in *Ovarian Malignancies*, p. 203. Edinburgh: Churchill Livingstone

Tazelaar, H.D., Bostwick, D.G., Ballon, S.C. *et al.* (1985) Conservative treatment of borderline ovarian tumors. *Obstet Gynecol* **66**, 417-22

Yoonessi, M., Crichard, K. and Celik, C. (1988) Borderline epithelial tumours of the ovary: ovarian intraepithelial neoplasia. *Obstet Gynecol Surv* **43**, 435-44

98 Which of the following features are found in gestational choriocarcinoma?

A) The majority of tumour cells are genetically XX.	FALSE
B) There is a poorer prognosis when it occurs after a term pregnancy.	TRUE
C) There is a poorer prognosis in older women.	FALSE
D) Metastatic disease may appear more than five years after the last conception.	TRUE
E) Metastases may show a villous structure.	FALSE

COMMENTS

Approximately half of all choriocarcinoma cases follow genetically normal pregnancies and slightly more than half of these are XY. Although hydatidiform moles are predominantly XX (both chromosomes usually being of paternal origin), some are heterozygous XY and this minority seem to be those with more malignant potential. There are few good cytogenetic studies on choriocarcinoma tissue but a predominance of XY has been reported.

Choriocarcinoma has a worse prognosis after term pregnancy, partly because of late diagnosis. Age is very important in the genesis of molar disease (the risk being twenty times greater in women over 45) but the response to treatment in older women is no worse than in young women.

Most of the malignant sequelae of hydatidiform mole occur within two years (the normal period of follow-up), but the appearance of choriocarcinoma many years after the last recorded pregnancy and in the postmenopausal period has been recorded on many occasions. Some of these cases may be unrecognised, non-gestational ovarian choriocarcinoma. Metastases which contain villi arise from invasive mole and have a tendency to regress spontaneously. Invasive mole rarely progresses to choriocarcinoma.

APPROPRIATE READING

Bagshawe, K.D. (1991) 'Trophoblastic tumors: diagnostic methods, epidemiology, clinical features and management' in M. Coppleson, J.M. Monaghan, P. Morrow and M.H. Tattersall (Eds) *Gynecologic Oncology* (2nd ed.), pp. 1027-43. Edinburgh: Churchill Livingstone

Paradinas, F.J. (1991) 'Pathology and classification of trophoblastic tumors' in M. Coppleson, J.M. Monaghan, P. Morrow and M.H. Tattersall (Eds) *Gynecologic Oncology* (2nd ed.), pp. 1013-26. Edinburgh: Churchill Livingstone

99 Regarding donor insemination (DI): since 1986 frozen semen has been used to reduce the risk of transmission of human immunodeficiency virus (HIV) by heterologous insemination. Which of the following statements are correct?

A) Decreased pregnancy rates occur with frozen sperm compared with fresh donation.   TRUE
B) Confirmation of ovulation is mandatory prior to commencing DI.   TRUE
C) Frozen semen is available for use after storage for three completed months.   FALSE
D) Intrauterine insemination is the treatment of choice following cervical cone biopsy whether using homologous or heterologous semen.   TRUE
E) Pregnancy rates obtained with frozen semen approximate to 10–15% per cycle.   TRUE

COMMENTS

Donor insemination is considered when infertility is due to azoospermia, severe oligospermia and for some couples following specialist genetic advice where there is an appreciable risk of an inherited disorder. The Human Fertilisation and Embryology (HF&E) Act was implemented in August 1991 and the Human Fertilisation and Embryology Authority established, whose principal task is to regulate by means of a licensing system research or treatment which involves the creation, storage and usage of human embryos, eggs and sperm. It maintains a code of practice and provides guidance to enable centres to achieve the objectives of the Act. The use of fresh semen for donor insemination is prohibited by the Act and only frozen semen that has been quarantined for six months may be used for the purpose.

Guidelines for the screening of gamete donors have been produced by the HFEA in co-operation with the Department of Health. Comparison of pregnancy rates achieved with fresh v. frozen sperm has suggested that decreased pregnancy rates occur with frozen sperm.

Three aspects require special attention: the treatment of associated factors, monitoring of semen sample quality and the timing of insemination. Each sample should contain = 20 million motile sperm at the time of insemination, and should have been screened for infection, e.g. *Chlamydia*. Insemination should be performed as close as possible to the time of ovulation. This may be determined by urinary LH testing in combination with basal body temperature recording and pelvic ultrasound. Insemination may be intracervical or intrauterine (IUI). Sperm are prepared for IUI either by a combination of wash-filtration using a medium, e.g. Earl's solution or the swim-up technique may be used. This facilitates harvesting the 'best' sperm separated from seminal plasma. Approximately 20–40 million motile sperms are used for each insemination and transferred into the uterine cavity using a catheter. With standard donor insemination a cumulative pregnancy rate of 40-50% may be expected with six cycles of treatment. To enhance fertility, superovulation techniques including IVF may be added. Careful monitoring to avoid ovarian hyperstimulation and high-order multiple births is mandatory.

APPROPRIATE READING

Barratt, C.C.R., Shanhan, M. and Cooke, I.D. (1990) Donor insemination – a look to the future. *Fertil Steril* **54**, 375-87

Human Fertilisation and Embryology Authority (1993) *Code of Practice* (revised ed.). London: HFEA

100 A depot preparation of a gonadotrophin releasing-hormone agonist (GnRHag):

A) Will immediately be associated with amenorrhoea.	FALSE
B) Will produce maximum shrinkage of uterine fibroids within three months.	TRUE
C) May produce endometrial atrophy within one month.	TRUE
D) Will always produce significant osteoporosis.	FALSE
E) Should never be adminstered in combination with other hormones.	FALSE

COMMENTS

The GnRH agonists initially stimulate the pituitary gland to produce increased gonadotrophin which in turn stimulates the ovaries. This means that the first implant is followed by a menstrual bleed. Down-regulation of the pituitary then leads to continuous suppression which is usually associated with amenorrhoea. Although breakthrough bleeding occurs in about 8% of subjects it is rarely heavy and thus many women receive relief from their menstrual problems. Suprisingly, in view of the initial stimulation of hormone output, the greatest rate of fibroid shrinkage is within the first month (West *et al.* 1987) and this is associated with endometrial ablation. The GnRH agonists lead to bone loss in some women who may lose 3-5% of their bone density. Whether this is likely to be clinically significant is open to debate as is the rate of recovery on stopping treatment. The hypo-oestrogenic side-effects, e.g. hot flushing, can be relieved by 'add back', i.e. giving a small dose of oestrogen in the form of HRT or a progestogen such as medroxy-progesterone acetate (West *et al.* 1992). However, it is not yet clear whether this will be sufficient to prevent the bone loss completely. A short course prior to hysterectomy has been shown to facilitate the ease of operation as well as providing symptom relief during the treatment period (Lumsden *et al.* 1987).

REFERENCES

Lumsden, M.A., West, C.P. and Baird, D.T. (1987) Goserelin therapy before surgery for uterine fibroids. *Lancet* **i**, 36-7

West, C.P., Lumsden, M.A., Lawson, S. *et al.* (1987) Shrinkage of uterine fibroids during therapy with Zoladex (ICI 118630) a luteinizing hormone releasing hormone agonist administered as a monthly subcutaneous depot. *Fertil Steril* **47**, 45

West, C.P., Lumsden, M.A., Hillier, H. *et al.* (1992) Potential role for medroxy progesterone acetate as an adjunct to goserelin (Zoladex) in the medical management of uterine fibroids. *Human Reprod* **7**, 328-332